In *A Simply Healthy Life*, Caroline Fau
Christian principles with practical wis
transformative guide to living intentic
every aspect of their lives. This book is a powerful reminder that
true health encompasses not only physical well-being but also
spiritual fulfillment and purposeful living.

KELLY LEVEQUE, founder of Be Well by Kelly

Sometimes starting healthy habits can feel overwhelming, but
Caroline Fausel's friendly tone helps the most habit-resisting
reader form a definition for a healthy life. I felt inspired to try
healthy habits I'd stopped and to try some I'd been too scared to
implement. Her challenges at the end of each chapter give the
reader focused energy toward implementing food, home, mental,
and relational practices that will give them a healthier, more
lasting life.

BAILEY T. HURLEY, author of *Together Is a Beautiful Place*

If you're looking for the ultimate guide to finding balance,
peace, and health in life, this book is for you! Caroline is great at
giving tangible advice on how to juggle all life's responsibilities
and challenges while remembering what is truly important.

MARY SMITH, owner of Mary's Whole Life and author of *Quick Prep
Paleo* and *Real Food Weeknights*

I have found that movement is so critical to my whole-body
health. I love how Caroline reframes exercise from being just a
gym to doing whatever movement you love to do. That will help
you keep moving your body in the long run!

TODD MCCULLOUGH, founder of TMAC Fitness

This book is an all-inclusive, accessible, actionable guide toward living your healthiest and happiest life. Whether you're looking for a total overhaul or to simply incorporate a few new habits—like mindset shifts, movement, or minimalism—Caroline gives you the blueprint to understand why it matters and how to integrate it into your life. This book can truly serve as a checklist for a life well lived—it's jam-packed with research, actionable suggestions, and helpful discussion topics to help you get there.

DANIKA BRYSHA, founder of Self-Care Society

In *A Simply Healthy Life*, Caroline Fausel teaches us to put self-care at the forefront of our busy lives. She outlines a simple formula that touches on many aspects of life, including how to find food that nourishes our bodies, how to free our homes from toxins, how to build meaningful friendships and lasting relationships, and best of all, how to create a life filled with intention, purpose, and faith. Caroline gently nudges us to create new habits and reminds us that it's never too late to change the course of our lives for the better. I, for one, am grateful for Caroline's loving advice, strong faith, and guiding wisdom, all of which shine through on every page of this book.

JENNY LEVINE FINKE, author of *Dear Gluten, It's Not Me, It's You*

Caroline has created the most thoughtful, encouraging, and informative road map to living your best and most fulfilled life! As a nutritionist, I really enjoyed the deep dive she offers on food and how food can truly act as medicine. And as a mom and a wife, I felt encouraged and supported as she walked through the other foundations of a happy, healthy, and fulfilled life. This is a must-read for everyone!

KATIE BRASWELL, MS, SPN, HTMA-P

A Simple Healthy Life is a must-read for anyone looking to make positive changes in their daily routine. Caroline provides practical tips on habit stacking to make healthy choices effortless, while also emphasizing the importance of nourishing your body with wholesome foods. This book is a game-changer for those seeking a more balanced and fulfilling life.

BLAIR HORTON, @holisticrendezvous

A Simply Healthy Life is an absolute must-have in your collection. Caroline's attention to detail makes my heart pitter-patter. From making simple, realistic goals and habits to creating your purpose and getting to the root of your new self, Caroline doesn't miss anything. Reading this book is like talking to a friend!

JENN BUMB, cookbook author and creator of Pretend It's a Donut

a SIMPLY
HEALTHY *life*

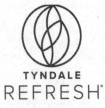

a SIMPLY HEALTHY *life*

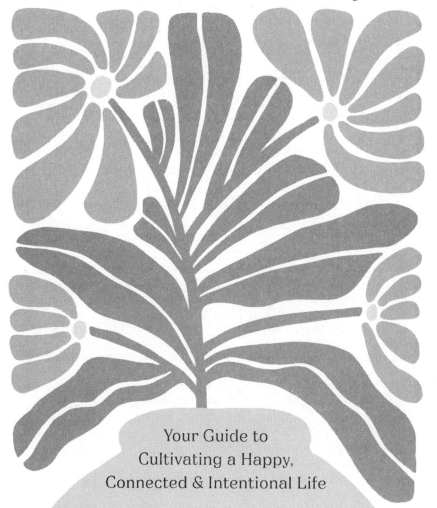

Your Guide to
Cultivating a Happy,
Connected & Intentional Life

CAROLINE FAUSEL

Visit Tyndale online at tyndale.com.

Visit the author online at oliveyouwhole.com.

Tyndale and Tyndale's quill logo are registered trademarks of Tyndale House Ministries. *Tyndale Refresh* and the Tyndale Refresh logo are trademarks of Tyndale House Ministries. Tyndale Refresh is a nonfiction imprint of Tyndale House Publishers, Carol Stream, Illinois.

A Simply Healthy Life: Your Guide to Cultivating a Happy, Connected, and Intentional Life

Cover designed by Libby Dykstra

Edited by Stephanie Rische

Published in association with the literary agency of WordServe Literary Group, www.wordserveliterary.com.

For information about special discounts for bulk purchases, please contact Tyndale House Publishers at csresponse@tyndale.com, or call 1-855-277-9400.

Library of Congress Cataloging-in-Publication Data

A catalog record for this book is available from the Library of Congress.

ISBN 978-1-4964-8690-5

Printed in the United States of America

30	29	28	27	26	25	24
7	6	5	4	3	2	1

This book is dedicated to my precious kiddos, Ella Rae and Owen. To me, you represent the future generation. Every day that we make healthy choices together, I'm encouraged that you will lead the charge to live a healthy lifestyle that will result in loving God, yourself, others, and the world. I always think I couldn't love you any more, and somehow, every day, I do! Keep being your joyful, encouraging, and genuine selves.

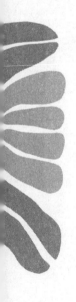

Contents

HEALTHY MADE EASY

When health is absent, wisdom cannot reveal itself,
art cannot manifest, strength cannot fight, wealth becomes
useless, and intelligence cannot be applied.
HEROPHILUS

If you're anything like me and the women I interact with every day, I have a hunch you want to be healthier and feel better. But there's so much conflicting information that bombards us, whether on social media, in ads, from friends and family, or in the health and wellness world. It's easy to become confused and stuck, not knowing which choice is best.

You might want to eat healthier, get to a healthy weight, and feel alive with energy, but you have absolutely zero idea of how to make that happen. Any time you try to research to make your dream a reality, you get overwhelmed by all the contradicting information.

Maybe you drag yourself through every day. You want to be able to keep up with your busy life or with your children. You want to finally feel good, without a list of lingering symptoms and ailments, but you're not sure what the underlying problem is, let alone how to solve it.

You might look around at the clutter in your home (or in the storage unit you pay for each month), and the idea of simplicity feels out of reach, only found on Pinterest or Instagram. Your soul craves a life with less chaos, but as you look at your kitchen island cluttered with mail and Goldfish crackers, you have no idea how to get there.

You might feel lonely and disconnected from community, but part of you is terrified by the prospect of diving into deep relationships. You made friends easily when you were a kid, but now initiating new relationships feels daunting. You're wondering where that village is that's supposed to be helping you.

Maybe you feel like there has to be more to life. You're longing for meaning and purpose, but it's hard to figure out what lights you up. You have a deep desire to grow closer to God, but you aren't sure where to even begin.

You might have young kids, and the days seem to blur together in an indistinguishable haze of dishes, laundry, errands, and meal prep. You worry you'll snap out of your motherhood trance when you drop your kids off at college, only to realize you have nothing left for yourself when they're gone. Or maybe you hustle so hard at work, and when the workday is done, you still find yourself working (or thinking about work). Your life is flying by, and all the ways you intend to care for yourself are on a future to-do list that never materializes.

Or maybe you're stuck in a life you don't love. You somehow ended up here, even though this isn't the career you wanted or the life you imagined. But you have no idea how to find your way to a new path.

In my health coaching sessions with women, I often start by asking, "What do you want for your life?" I'm often met with tear-filled eyes. Many people have buried their dreams long ago, or they haven't allowed themselves to dream in the first place.

It's easy to fall into automated routines just to get through our (very) busy days. With our lives going about a million miles an hour, it can be hard to take even an hour to ourselves to answer the question "What do I really want?" But here's the thing: without making a plan and intentional choices, we're unlikely to live the life of purpose we desire.

How about you? Have you taken the time to sit with this question of what you want for your life? Maybe you've never given yourself permission to really get to the deeper answer. Or maybe you know the answer, but you're scared to pursue it because it will rock the boat.

You may find yourself daydreaming of a new venture that won't stop tugging at your heart, but you already have too much on your plate. Or you may be thinking, *I'm way too busy taking care of everyone else to invest in myself.* But it doesn't have to be this way. We are designed to live a full, healthy life—in heart, mind, body, and soul. We can care for others best when we are filled up ourselves.

What Whole-Person Wellness Looks Like

I believe wellness is inherently holistic—it involves the connection between body, mind, and soul. When it comes to the medical realm, people tend to assume their symptoms have only a physical cause. And in the church, people may be encouraged to focus only on the spiritual. But in reality, humans are integrated beings. If we're not moving our bodies, we often feel stuck in our faith and our relationships. If we're thriving in our faith, it can help us thrive in other areas too. When we're fueling our bodies as they were designed to be, we feel more alive, and that energy sparks just about every other area of our lives.

This is how *The Message* captures 1 Corinthians 3:16-17: "You realize, don't you, that you are the temple of God, and God himself is present in you? No one will get by with vandalizing God's temple, you can be sure of that. God's temple is sacred—and you, remember, *are* the temple." No matter what worldview you're coming from, I think we can all agree that humans are awe inspiring. I believe that we are all created in the image of God. This belief is at the heart of my own health and wellness journey—I want to live with vitality and energy so I can live out my God-given purpose with as much impact as possible.

When I'm talking to Christian women about focusing on their own health, wellness, and relationships, I often get pushback. I've even heard people argue that "self-care is selfish." It's true that a meaningful life includes pouring into others and using our gifts for good. But we aren't meant to live on empty.

No matter where we are in terms of our faith journey, none of us are able to serve others well unless we're also caring for ourselves. Unfortunately, our faith communities don't always encourage this balance. In fact, some of the drive we feel to do and be everything to everyone else comes from within the church. But the destructive belief that we should ignore our own needs isn't from Scripture.

In Christian culture, there's a tendency to idolize a martyr mentality—we're taught that ignoring our own needs and wants is the path to holiness. But when Jesus gave the Greatest Commandment, he said we are to love our neighbor as ourselves (see Matthew 22:39). This implies a baseline of caring for our own needs. When we receive God's love and care, we can serve others out of that overflow. When we focus on everyone else's needs except our own, it is an entirely unsustainable lifestyle. We are left exhausted both physically and emotionally, and most likely bitter and resentful.

Jesus himself gave us an example of taking time to himself (gasp!) so he could be filled with his Father's love *before* he went into the crowds and poured out that love. Here's one of many examples in Scripture: "Very early in the morning, while it was still dark, Jesus got up, left the house and went off to a solitary place, where he prayed" (Mark 1:35). Jesus regularly removed himself from the chaos and the needs of the people around him to be with his Father. What I find so fascinating about this is that Jesus was fully human and fully God. He and God were one, but he still needed to set aside time to recharge and reset so he could be fully present and fulfill his calling.

"Sure," you might be saying, "but he wasn't giving himself a mani-pedi—he was praying!" I get it, but the point is that he took a break from caring for other people so he could be filled up before he poured out. (Also, there's more to self-care than a day at the spa, but we'll get to that later.)

When you are intentional about what matters most to you, you'll be a better friend, wife, mom, executive, or fill-in-the-blank. When you are filled up first, you will have the reserves to do the things that God has called you to. You'll soon find that self-care is a way to show love not only to yourself but also to the people around you.

When you prioritize your health and wellness, your spiritual formation, your relationships with friends and family, and God's purpose for your life, you will be able to flourish—and help those you love flourish too.

My Journey to Wellness

As I'll share about later in this book, I was often sick as a child. A slew of unknown food intolerances combined with frequent antibiotic use led me to suffer from significant digestive issues. My stomach hurt nearly every night, and no one seemed to have answers. This lack of control about my body turned me toward health and wellness from a young age.

It wasn't until I was an adult and my husband, Chaz, and I had our little girl, Ella Rae, that I realized food can be medicine. If I ate clean, anti-inflammatory foods, I experienced zero stomachaches. Not only that, but I had more energy than ever before (and keep in mind, I had a one-year-old!).

When I found a way of eating that worked for my family, I wanted to share it with the world. That's how my company, Olive You Whole, was born. This was my mission: "I help you build a healthy, connected, intentional life that fulfills your greatest purpose," and that mission has never wavered. I love creating resources and recipes to help people live a simply healthy life. My passion to help people on this journey also led me to become a certified health and wellness coach. This book is another avenue for me to share what I've learned along the way (often the hard way!).

Don't Let Life Choose for You

My hope is that reading this book will be like having a health coach in your pocket (or your crossbody bag or whatever you fancy!). I want to help you envision the life of your dreams and give you both the information and the tools to be able to achieve it. Little by little, thought by thought and habit by habit, you will begin to change your life.

Living intentionally includes both having a long-term plan and making intentional, on-purpose choices toward that goal every day. Either you will make choices about how you want your life to go and the legacy you want to leave, or life will choose for you.

As a health coach and wellness expert, I think of a thriving life being healthy in the most comprehensive sense of the word. It's another way of saying you're functioning at your prime. When it comes to your body, this means your systems are all functioning optimally. You're fueling your body in a way that meets its needs, which results in you feeling energetic, refreshed, happy, and thriving. When it comes to your environment, being healthy means cultivating a fresh, clean, life-giving home. The simplicity of your surroundings reflects an inner sense of peace. Your shopping choices make a positive impact on your community and the world. When it comes to relationships and community, being healthy means having friends who allow you to be the fullest and most genuine expression of yourself. It means having relationships in which you are free to both love and be loved. When it comes to your spiritual life, being healthy means you're able to pursue your connection with God and practice spiritual disciplines. When you're healthy, you feel alive as you live out the unique purpose God has called you to.

> Either you will make choices about how you want your life to go and the legacy you want to leave, or life will choose for you.

Creating a Strong Foundation

Over the past decade, I've focused personally and professionally on living intentionally in four areas: health and wellness, environment, relationships, and faith. In my training to become a health coach, I learned that all these areas make up the roots of the functional wellness tree. When you're healthy in these areas, you will be able to lead a fulfilling life and pursue your goals and dreams. You will also create a healthy foundation so you can live with vitality and avoid future disease.

In each chapter, we'll focus on the essentials, clearing away the clutter so you can make the choices that are best for you and your family. Each chapter ends with three levels of challenges so you can put this new knowledge to work right away.

Through these chapters, I want to empower you to do the following:

- build healthy habits and sustainable patterns
- eat in a way that makes you feel alive
- find a movement pattern that you love that gives your body energy
- free your body from harmful toxins
- create a healthy, simple, and inviting home environment that brings you joy
- manage your stuff so your stuff doesn't manage you
- take inventory of your thoughts and become more optimistic toward yourself and others
- find community and build healthy, uplifting friendships
- foster healthy, loving relationships and patterns within your family
- rest so you feel rejuvenated and able to love and serve others
- feel fulfilled by what you do

A healthy life starts with getting intentional. Making deliberate choices in these areas has made the greatest influence on my life—and I think it can do the same for you.

How to Use This Book

Every day we make about 35,000 choices. Many of these choices may seem insignificant, but when they're added together, they make a dramatic impact. When we steer our choices in the direction we want, life won't just happen to us. We'll live the life we were meant to live—a healthy, intentional life.

With all the information bombarding us, it can be hard to cut through all the noise to get to what's most important and most actionable. In this book, I've tried to give you the lightning bolt version of what I've learned over the past twelve years in the health and wellness industry. In each chapter, I'll help you determine what's worth prioritizing and what's best to let go of. You'll learn how to create lasting change and how to cultivate habits so you can slowly but surely put everything into practice.

There are a lot of suggestions in this book! You might read it cover to cover and then come back to specific sections as you're ready to tackle them. Or you can look at the chapter titles and decide which topic to focus on first. After reading the chapter, you can choose one of the challenges at the end and focus on it for thirty days. Once you've gotten a handle on that, you can move on to the next-level challenge or move on to another chapter.

The way you use this book is up to you, but know that every suggestion is invitational. Don't feel pressured to make every idea a reality if it doesn't work for you or for this particular season. No matter where you are on this journey toward a simply healthy life, the goal is to keep growing, one step at a time.

PART ONE

Health and Wellness

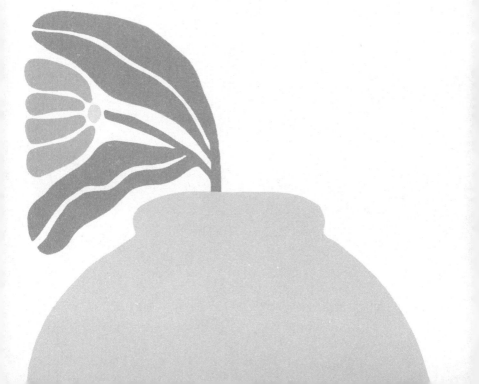

CHAPTER 1

CHANGING YOUR LIFE FOR GOOD

Our thoughts become our words, our words become our beliefs,
our beliefs become our habits, and our habits become our realities.

JEN SINCERO

When it comes to health, we want change, and we want it *now*. We want the fairy-tale ending that takes zero work to get there. Unfortunately, that's just not how it goes down. We know we need discipline. But how can we be disciplined in so many areas at once?

It comes down to two things: goals and habits.

When we think about forming new habits, we often relegate this process to New Year's resolutions or expensive new gym memberships. But we can form new goals and habits absolutely any time!

Whether we realize it or not, our days are already made up of habits—some of them intentional and others we don't even think about. In this chapter, we'll lay the foundation for creating habits and making them stick. We'll start with one habit at a time, and then you can use this strategy to create lifelong habits in other areas of your life as well.

Making Goals That Stick

If you want to change your life, the key is to make one choice at a time. You may have a massive dream, but every dream is built by small, quick wins that eventually add up to a big change. These step-by-step gains are like the first pebbles falling off a snowy mountain that, while initially tiny, eventually cause an avalanche.

In order to turn your big vision into small, achievable steps, you'll need SMART goals: specific, measurable, attainable, relevant, and time-bound.[1]

Let's say you have a goal to walk a certain number of steps every day for three months. A habit that might accompany that goal would be to consistently take the stairs instead of the elevator. Both your goals and your habits work together toward the same larger goal—in this case, being more active.

Specific means your goal is clear and precise. The reality is, a vague goal likely will not get accomplished. As you set your goal, you'll want to ask yourself questions like "What?," "When?," "Where?," and "How?"

Measurable means you have a clear way to define success. What metrics will let you know the goal is complete? The questions to ask here are "How much?" or "How many?"

Attainable means you can achieve this goal. Given your life stage, health, level of fitness, work and family situation, and time constraints, is this goal possible for you in this season?

Magic Wand Exercise

When a new client comes to me for health coaching, one of the first things we do is the Magic Wand exercise. Let's do it together now! Get out your journal or a piece of paper, and answer this question: If you could wave a magic wand and your life, family, and health could be exactly as you wanted them to be, what would that look like?

Use a stream-of-consciousness style of writing. Don't edit as you go—just write what you're thinking. Try to be as detailed as possible. Where do you live? How do you feel every day? What's your financial situation? What are your relationships like?

Now it's time to take inventory of your life as it is right now. You can start by going to oliveyouwhole.com/inventory and ranking different areas of your life from 0 to 10. What surprised you? Were there any categories that were higher or lower than you expected?

Relevant means this goal is in line with your values, your life purpose, and the direction you want to go. You can refer to the Magic Wand exercise to gain clarity about this.

Time-bound means your goal has a beginning and an end, and the time period has been decided in advance. When you put dates around your goal, it helps you get prepared and focus during this specific window.

Once you've decided on a SMART goal, write it down somewhere you will see it often. Anticipate setbacks, and have a plan in place to keep going when you hit these speed bumps. This knowledge that setbacks are part of the process will keep you going even when hiccups come along. Also keep in mind that your goals will evolve over time, so don't be afraid to make changes as necessary. Consider finding an accountability buddy or working with a coach to keep you on track as you work toward your goals.

As you achieve your goals, one at a time, you will eventually begin to change your life. Each small victory draws you closer to your long-term goals. And as habits become automatic, they will continue long after your goal has been accomplished.

Why Habits?

Our brains are encouraged to create habits because we're lazy. Seriously! Habits take something that would otherwise take a lot of processing power and simplify it by making it automatic. It's kind of like my kids on the first snow of the season. They all bundle up until they look like the Michelin man and head to our favorite sledding hill, pulling their sleds with their friends behind them. The surface of the snow is completely smooth, except for some bunny prints here and there.

At this point, one of my kids has to volunteer to go first. Doesn't every kid want to go first? Usually—but not with sledding. Why not? Because when their sled sits on top of the freshly fallen snow, they have to scoot. And scoot. And scoot. It's not a fast, smooth, fun ride to the bottom. The path is paved with endurance, with the promise that the effort will eventually be worth it.

Our brains' neural pathways work in a similar way. When we're forming a new habit, it's like creating the sledding path. It's hard. It takes a lot of work. But when we stick with it, it eventually becomes a habit—something we can do without thinking about it.

It's tempting to think of habits as grand acts of discipline that other people (not you) do, like your friend who runs six miles every morning—rain, shine, or snow. But even if you don't feel like a particularly disciplined person, you still have plenty of habits. In fact, 45 percent of our daily behaviors are made up of habits.[2]

Think of the things you do the same way every day—making your coffee, choosing the spot you sit for breakfast, checking your email, packing your bag for work. So much of what we do is habitual, because habits make our lives easier.

Whether you realize it or not, the things you do over and over are essentially building the person you are. Habits affect what you think about and how you talk to yourself. Habits affect what you eat and when you eat. Habits affect your morning routine, the way you move your body, your nightly routine, and when you go to bed. When you tweak these habits to make them healthier, you can change your life!

Forming a New Habit

If habits sound rather mundane to you, I have some exciting news. We can use the science of habit formation and behavior change to help us *mindlessly* become the people we hope to become. That's pretty amazing! Likewise, Scripture talks about how our character is often built in small, daily acts. It says in 1 Corinthians 10:31, "Whether you eat or drink, or whatever you do, do all to the glory of God" (ESV). Little by little, we are being sanctified and becoming more like Christ. More often than not, those changes happen through the intentional habits we cultivate.

In his book *Atomic Habits*, author James Clear describes the four stages of habit: cue, craving, response, and reward.[3] This four-step process happens every time you perform a habit. If you want to analyze your current habits, create new habits, or break bad habits, it's important to understand this process.

A cue is what sparks you to perform the habit, such as putting your Bible and journal on your coffee table to cue you to spend time with Jesus when you wake up. Craving is the second step. In this stage, you're desiring the reward on the other side of the habit. If you're a runner, although you might enjoy the run itself, the craving could be the endorphin rush or "runner's high" you experience. Response is the habit that you're performing, whether it's a thought or an action. The reward is the goal of every habit, and each of the previous three steps are in pursuit of this reward. Our brains are constantly scanning for rewards, trying to create more habit loops to simplify and automate our lives.

The reason we can form new habits and new ways of being is because of the brain's capacity for neuroplasticity—the ability to change connections and behavior in response to stimulation or information. This allows us to learn new things and create new pathways in our brains (like new habits!).[4]

Use Blatant Reminders

Make the cue for your new habit so obvious that you practically have to do it. You can set up your environment to help make this happen. I've heard of people who want to read their Bible daily putting it on the floor by their bed, so when they wake up and get out of bed, they would literally have to walk over their Bible or move it out of the way if they didn't want to read it. You could also put healthy foods in the cabinet where you typically go when you're reaching for a snack, or you could set an alarm on your phone for several times throughout the day as a reminder to stand up and stretch.

Consider Habit Stacking

Since so much of our life is already filled with habits, we can use the existing habits to our advantage! One strategy for creating a cue is called habit stacking—adding your new habit on top of another one that's already cemented in your routine. For example, maybe you want to start applying a night cream before bed. You could add this on to a habit that you already do consistently, like brushing your teeth. So immediately after brushing your teeth, you would apply night cream. Or if you want to start changing your thought patterns, each time you wash your hands throughout your day, you could look in the mirror and say something positive or practice a moment of gratitude. Adding on a new habit to an already solid habit increases the likelihood that your new habit will stick.

Implement Delayed Gratification

My husband, Chaz, doesn't get annoyed by much. But he recently shared with me that he was frustrated that when I made my espresso drink in the morning, I failed to dump the beans into the compost and clean out the portafilter. Since I usually make my coffee first, he had to dump it out and clean it before he could make his own drink.

I could see how annoying this was for him, and I really wanted to change. So I used my craving, which was to drink a delicious latte, to form my new habit. I told myself that I couldn't drink my coffee until I'd cleaned out my portafilter. Even though cleaning isn't typically a strength of mine, it worked, because my craving for good coffee was strong enough!

If there's something you don't want to do (such as making your bed in the morning), pair it with something you enjoy (such as starting the diffuser with your favorite essential oil blend so your room smells lovely all day).

Start Tiny

This might seem obvious, but is this habit even possible for you? If I want my habit to be to run ten miles every day, I might be able to do that eventually. But could I do that consistently starting today? No, I could not. The first rule of habits is to make sure this habit is attainable in the first place.

BJ Fogg shares the "five ability factors": time, money, physical effort,

CHANGING YOUR LIFE FOR GOOD

mental effort, and routine. Do you have enough time, money, physical capability, and mental energy to do this behavior? And does this behavior fit into your current routine, or do you need to make adjustments for it to work?[5] These are critical questions to ask, because they help you determine whether your habit is feasible or not. You don't want to set a goal that you're not capable of achieving.

When a task is massive, we have to rely on our motivation and willpower to make it happen. I don't know about you, but for me, motivation can be a fickle friend. We may start out with lots of ambition, but it's not long before that energy wanes. This may seem counterintuitive, but the way to achieve big goals is to break each goal into steps that are so tiny we don't need much motivation or willpower to complete them.

Ashley, a health coaching client of mine, shared with me that she had worked with health coaches in the past, but it had never worked out for her. She wanted to accomplish massive goals, like cooking everything she ate entirely from scratch, but she struggled to stick with these goals. When we sat down to create her first goal, she suggested that she stop eating out entirely. At the time, she was eating out once a week for lunch and almost every evening for dinner. Given that she'd struggled with accomplishing similar big goals in the past, we worked together to pare down her big goal to a smaller goal of not eating out only at lunchtime. This felt like a more manageable goal and provided her with an easy win after our first week of working together. This victory propelled her toward bigger goals and continued success.

So the goal isn't to run a marathon. That might be the end goal, but when you get started, this isn't what you're working toward (remember, we're thinking tiny here!). At first, the goal might be to just put on your tennis shoes. Maybe you'll end up walking, maybe you'll run for a little bit, or maybe you'll just put your shoes on and think about it. That's okay—we're talking about baby steps here.

Continue to ask yourself, *Could this goal be any tinier?* until the answer is no. Now *that* is your tiny habit. Once you make this small thing a habit, it becomes easier to add to it.

As you complete your new habit over and over again, you begin to trust that you are, in fact, capable of change. Your success leads to more success. You realize that you can do hard things!

Remove Barriers

One way to make your new habit attainable is to remove anything that's in the way.

Chaz and I divide up the house chores, including the dishes. I load the dishes throughout the day, and he loads them after dinner, starts the dishwasher, and unloads the dishwasher in the morning. When we were doing our yearly check-in on our anniversary trip, it became clear that I wasn't keeping my end of our dish duties. I'm an Enneagram 7, and I don't love mundane things, so the dishes were piling up on the counters and in the sink. Chaz and I took a step back and thought about how we could ensure that this task got done. I remembered that my friend Alissa's kids put their dishes in the dishwasher after every meal and snack, and I thought, *Well, why can't our kids do that too?*

Then we asked ourselves, *Are there any barriers that are getting in the way of making this goal happen? What can we do about those barriers?*

We realized our barrier was that Owen, who was six years old at the time, couldn't reach the sink to rinse off his dishes before putting them in the dishwasher. There was an easy solution for this—we ordered a stool that would be there by the time we got home! Now our kiddos know the expectation, and they load their own dishes in the dishwasher. This may seem like a simple example, but the principle applies to larger problems as well.

Tiny Habits for Massive Goals

- Run a marathon: put on your running shoes
- Make yourself breakfast: take out the carton of eggs (or another ingredient)
- Get eight hours of sleep: get in bed at 10 p.m.
- Read one book a month: read one page at night
- Stay well hydrated: pour yourself one glass of water in the morning
- Tidy your kitchen every night: put one dish in the dishwasher
- Lower your stress: pray or meditate for thirty seconds after waking up

Treat Yourself

The reward is why we're doing the habit in the first place. Be sure that the reward is something you're really excited about. If it's not attractive enough, the habit loop will fail, and your habit won't stick.

What works for me is to take something I already want and delay my gratification until I complete the habit. For example, I had a goal of using the squeegee to clean our glass shower walls after taking a shower. It keeps the glass clean for longer and removes the dried water droplets, but since it's a mundane task, I'm not naturally inclined to do it consistently. To motivate myself, I tell myself that I don't get my warm, dry towel until I squeegee the shower walls. Each person's rewards are different (the reward of a clean shower may be enough for some people, like Chaz!), but experiment until you find something that makes sense for you.

Get Back on the Horse

Studies show that missing a day doesn't cause the habit to fail forever, but you want it to be more common to do the habit than not do it.[6] If you skip one day, the habit is likely still ingrained. But missing more than one day in a row makes it seem like skipping is the easier path forward. Track your habits, and try to be as consistent as possible. If you miss a day, recommit yourself to your goal. The faster you get back on the horse, the more likely you'll be successful in the long term with your new habit.

Choosing Your Habit

Forming new habits has everything to do with our identity. As author Jen Sincero says, "Identities come equipped with matching habits."[7] Habits are often aspirational, because the whole point is the desire to become a better version of ourselves. The most successful habits are formed when we buy into the habit as part of our new identity.

I recently decided I wanted to start running again. I ran cross-country in high school, and running was my biggest form of exercise in college, even when I didn't have to anymore. But when I had Ella Rae, it became harder to run. Either I'd have to run with a stroller or find childcare. But with both my kids in elementary school, it seemed like a good time to pick up this hobby again.

I knew that in order to make this habit stick, I had to make it identity based. I wouldn't keep up with it if my mentality was, *Oh, I'm not a runner, I just run occasionally.* Instead, I told Chaz that I was going to start identifying as a runner. Being a runner means I go on runs often. It means I like running, and I will even run on vacation!

> Forming new habits is fun because it's like deciding who you're going to be in the future.

Forming new habits is fun because it's like deciding who you're going to be in the future. The first step is to believe that becoming that person is possible. You can decide now that you already *are* that person. That belief will fuel your ability to stick with the habits that reflect the new you.

As you begin thinking about choosing which habits you want to build into your life, it's important to start with the end in mind. What are you working toward, and why is that important to you? Maybe you want to get better sleep. But you don't want to get better sleep for kicks and giggles—you probably want to get better sleep so you have more energy for yourself, your spouse, your kids, or your friends. And why is that important to you? Maybe it's because as a tired, frazzled version of yourself, you feel like you're not showing up the way you want to and instead of showing love to others, you yell and lose your patience. Now *that* is your true motivation—your *why* for prioritizing sleep.

Write your why on a sticky note and put it somewhere you'll see it multiple times a day to keep you on track.

High-Yield Habits

When my clients hire me as a health coach, they often have a particular reason—one area that feels most crucial to focus on. Maybe that's true

High-Yield Habit Exercise

When it comes to change, we're often clear on the problem but hazy on possible solutions. Without committing to any specific action or habit, let's just get some ideas out on paper.

Grab your journal or a piece of paper. At the top of the page, write the area you want to focus on. Then set a timer for five minutes, and write down as many different solutions (behaviors) for your problem as possible. Don't edit as you go—just write, write, write!

Next, set your timer for ten minutes. Do a little research about what the experts are saying about your problem and add those ideas to your list.

Draw a horizontal line and a vertical line to divide your paper into four quadrants. At the top of the vertical line, write, "Very effective at helping me." At the bottom of the vertical line, write, "Not very effective at helping me." On the left side of the horizontal line, write, "No, I can't get myself to do this behavior." On the right side of the horizontal line, write, "Yes, I can get myself to do this behavior."

Now look at each of the behaviors you brainstormed and find a place for them in one of the four quadrants, taking into consideration how impactful this behavior would be to help solve your problem or accomplish your dream, and how motivated you are to do this behavior.

After mapping every behavior, zoom out and look at the entire chart. The behaviors in the top right are the ones that are highly impactful and that you're motivated to do. These are called high-yield habits. When you're choosing your first habit to try to form, choose one in the top right quadrant.[8]

High-Yield Habit Chart

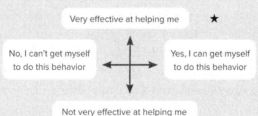

Habits That Have Positive Ripple Effects

- Regular exercise
- Positive morning routine
- Healthy sleep hygiene
- Getting enough sleep

- Stretching
- Cooking at home
- Keeping a food journal
- Meal prepping
- Making your bed

- Journaling
- Reading
- Prayer
- Tracking expenses
- Practicing gratitude[9]

for you too. Maybe you're experiencing significant stress, having trouble sleeping, feeling a lack of energy, struggling with digestive issues, or feeling lonely.

Choose just one area to focus on for now (but don't worry—you can use this process with other areas once you've mastered this one). Once you've chosen the issue you'd like to address, complete the High-Yield Habit exercise.

Breaking Bad Habits

Habit formation isn't just about creating positive new habits. It's also about breaking bad habits. Just as we thought through why we wanted to start a new habit, it's crucial to figure out why we keep coming back to a bad habit. Usually we can look at the reward of the habit for a clue about why we're doing it in the first place.

The key to breaking a bad habit is essentially the opposite of how we form a good habit, and it revolves around the habit loop. For the cue, make it invisible. For the craving, make it unattractive. For the response, make it difficult. For the reward, make it unsatisfying.[10] We're most likely to experience success in breaking a bad habit if we keep the reward and swap out the bad behavior for a good behavior.

Let's take the example of social media. If I were to ask you how much time you spend on social media, you might estimate about an hour a day. Then you look at your screen time report and realize it's actually closer to four hours a day! I'm guessing that if you mapped out how you want to spend your time, spending hours on social media wouldn't make the list.

This is a problem for most of us. And while we might claim that social media makes us feel connected to our friends, in reality, we scroll social media because we're bored, we're avoiding another task, or it's an ingrained habit.

If you want to quit any habit, including mindless scrolling, the first thing you need to do is figure out *why* you're doing it. There may be lots of different reasons, so try to be really honest with yourself and get to the root of it. Once you've nailed this down, don't just try to break the habit cold turkey—find a way to get the same benefit or reward from a different habit. If you determine the underlying reason for your scrolling is boredom, you could replace that habit by bringing a book in your purse to read when you get bored. If you discover you're doing it out of loneliness, you could call a friend instead.

As you reflect on the reason you engage in a bad habit, you may realize it's because you need better coping skills. If this is you, you are not alone! Almost everyone has some unhealthy coping patterns. The key is to recognize them so we can be intentional about making a change.

The first question to ask yourself is, *How am I feeling when I engage in this negative behavior?* Are you doing this because you're bored? Sad? Angry?

The second question to ask yourself is, *How can I swap this negative behavior with a positive new habit?*

Many people use food as a coping mechanism. Maybe you feel sad one night, and you eat an entire sleeve of Girl Scout Cookies. Your stomach may regret it later, but there's the immediate reward of receiving comfort and avoiding sadness while the Thin Mints hit your taste buds. If you *always* eat a sleeve of Girl Scout Cookies when you're sad, this becomes ingrained as a habit. To switch this habit, brainstorm positive coping strategies that could bring you comfort. For example, when you're feeling sad, you might call a friend, drink warm tea, take an Epsom salt bath, go to an infrared sauna, read a book, write in your journal, or go for a walk.

Rule of Life

When you're working on changing your lifestyle through habits, it's too overwhelming to set twenty goals and try to work on them all at once. This is why New Year's resolutions often fail: it's impossible to prioritize so many areas of your life simultaneously. The key to keeping momentum is to add just one new habit at a time. As you continue in this lifestyle of making wise choices, you'll be able to stack more habits on top of one another. This is the slow, steady process of building a healthy lifestyle.

John Mark Comer calls this kind of intentional habit stacking a Rule of Life. He defines it as "a schedule and set of practices and relational rhythms that create space for us to be with Jesus, become like him, and do as he did, as we live in alignment with our deepest desires."[11]

Rules are essentially habits that keep our lives and our actions integrated with what we say is important to us. Sometimes we *think* something is important to us, but when we take inventory of our actions, they don't align with that value.

Developing a rule of life gives us the structure we need to stay aligned with our values. Which habits are in line with your values? These are the habits you want to keep. Which habits aren't contributing to who you want to become? These are the habits you want to break. Are there new habits you want to adopt?

Your rule of life is all about rhythms. What rhythms do you want to create in terms of your health, your environment, your relationships, and your faith? What habits can you cultivate—daily, weekly, monthly, and annually—that promote what is most important to you?

These habits aren't set in stone. I recommend that you revisit them regularly to see how they're working for you and find out what needs to be tweaked. This rule should be life giving, not restrictive.

When we start small, with a tiny habit, we are able to achieve small wins. Those small wins give us the momentum to continue forming new habits for self-improvement. As we continue to evaluate and modify our habits, we build a healthy lifestyle and eventually become who we want to be.

Habits Challenge

Beginner challenge: Choose one new habit to practice for thirty days. Remember to make your habit specific. What is your goal, broken into small steps? When and where will you do this task? How will you measure it? Why are you passionate about creating this habit?

Intermediate challenge: Choose one habit you want to break. Do some soul searching to determine the deeper reason you keep coming back to this habit. Then replace that behavior with a healthy habit that fulfills the same reward or longing.

Advanced challenge: Create a rule of life using the worksheet at oliveyouwhole.com/rule-of-life. This exercise will help you create a holistic plan to develop healthy habits in different areas in your life.

CHAPTER 2

FOOD AS THE CULPRIT
AND THE CURE

Eat food. Not too much. Mostly plants.
MICHAEL POLLAN

For most people, food is packed with emotion. I know that's true for me!
When I was young, I would go to my maternal grandmother's house for
the sole purpose of making banana bread, and to this day, the smell of
banana bread reminds me how important family is. Now when I bake
with my kiddos, I know they're creating fond memories too. I remember
walking into the kitchen every morning during my childhood to see
my dad doing his devotions while eating frosted shredded wheat with
banana slices on top. When I eat a banana for breakfast, I feel a wave
of appreciation for his neverending dedication to his faith. Maybe there
are specific foods you make that remind you of certain holidays, snacks
you always eat on a road trip, or treats you reach for when you're sad
(Ben and Jerry's anyone?).

So when we talk about the foods that fuel our bodies best, it's natural
for this to bring up an emotional reaction. Maybe you have zero desire
to change the foods you're eating, or you may feel defensive about your

eating habits. But after you read about how different foods can positively affect how you feel, you just might be willing to give this healthy eating thing a shot!

We don't typically think of food in terms of medicine, but food can be both the culprit for symptoms we're experiencing *and* the cure for what ails us. The food you're eating could be contributing to negative symptoms you're experiencing, but it can also be a tool to heal those same symptoms. I know, because I have experienced both myself.

When I was growing up, I was a pretty unhealthy child. Let me pause here and tell you that I have the best parents in the world—truly. They loved me and they did their best, but knowledge about food and nutrition in the nineties just wasn't what it is today. Let's be real—as kids, we were squirting Easy Cheese directly into our mouths. What could possibly have gone wrong?

I remember after dinner every night, I would tell my mom that my tummy hurt. Every. Single. Night. She didn't know what could be causing the problem. Back then, there wasn't talk about food intolerances. You either had a true allergy (like my sister's allergy to peanuts, which landed her a spot at the "peanut-free table") or you didn't. There was no in-between.

My digestive issues got so bad that I ended up missing a lot of fourth grade. My friend Katie would bring my work to me almost every day after school. My mom took me to many specialists to figure out what was going on, but I don't remember a single doctor asking what I was eating. Doesn't that just blow your mind? They'd do a scope or two and then send me home, saying, "She'll be fine." In addition to my digestive issues, I got sick so often that from a young age, I started asking for Z-Paks instead of the disgusting bubblegum liquid.

I didn't have a chronic illness as a child. I didn't have a traumatic surgery or a long stint in the hospital. But my body did feel out of control. I didn't have a single answer about my health. I didn't know why I kept getting sick. I didn't know why sometimes my stomach hurt and other times it felt fine. I felt like I was walking on a field covered with land mines, never knowing when one would be set off and I'd feel sick again.

I first started hearing about healthy eating from Rhonda, my best friend Amy Beth's mom. While I've known Amy Beth since the womb (our parents were friends from church), we were reunited in sixth grade when we attended the same middle school. Rhonda was a nutritionist, and I would go to their house and literally sit at Rhonda's feet. "White bread is made from ultra-processed flour? Wait, sugar is bad for you?"

The more she shared and the more I continued to learn on my own, the more I realized that it *was* possible to have a level of control over my health. The things I put in my body affected how I felt, both daily and systemically. Thus began my journey to healthy eating (though it wasn't without its ups and downs along the way).

What Should We Eat?

This desire to live my healthiest life led me to become a vegetarian in college. I had been a vegetarian for about a year in third grade, but mainly because my friend Erica was too, so why not? But let's be honest, I was the pizza-and-donuts kind of vegetarian, not the kale-and-beets kind.

Back to college: I heard somewhere that pork wasn't great for you, so I cut it out of my diet. When it came time for me to study abroad in Cortona, Italy, I checked the "vegetarian" box for our nightly group dinners. Just think about all those Italian meats—pepperoni, prosciutto, pancetta—they're *all* pork. I didn't go back to eating meat for four years!

Incidentally, that same summer, my now-husband, Chaz, was a morning cook at a Young Life camp, frying up *hundreds* of pounds of meat at once. Seeing that much meat at once was enough to cause him to go vegetarian too!

When we got married, our "plan" (can you read the irony there?) to have our first child eight years later ended after six *weeks* when we got pregnant with Ella Rae. I was just twenty-two years old. Like Olaf from *Frozen*, we figured that eight years from our wedding, we'd be responsible adults with lots of wealth and wisdom. Instead, we were babies having babies. And as fresh-out-of-college babies, what did we *not* have? Money.

Chaz was in his third year of medical school when Ella Rae was born. So not only was he not bringing in money yet, we were paying for him to be in medical school. My degree in graphic design landed me a job for a measly $25,000 a year. When I was pregnant, we qualified for every government subsidy. That included food stamps and a program called WIC (which stands for women, infants, and children). Unlike food stamps, which was just a certain amount of money loaded onto a debit card, WIC provided coupons for specific grocery items.

As a precursor to being a part of this program, I was required to attend a government-mandated nutrition class provided by the WIC program. I was shocked by what they provided as "up-to-date" nutrition information and what items were deemed crucial for women, infants, and children. At one point the teacher asked us to participate in a call-and-response about milk. She said, "What kind of dairy should you get?" And we were to call back, "Fat free!"

Even at that point in my health journey, I knew that fat is *the* most redeeming quality of dairy! We were allotted a gallon of fat-free milk a week, plus one-pound blocks of fat-free cheese. We were also allotted loaves of bread and boxes of cereal. Although we could get fruits and vegetables, the limit was ten dollars a month. A *month*!

When Ella Rae was born prematurely at thirty weeks, we were quickly thrown into the unknown world of parenting. When it was time for Ella Rae to eat solids, I had a full-blown nutritional crisis. It's one thing to make nutritional choices for yourself; it's a whole other ball game when you're making them for your child.

Chaz and I were still nearly vegan at the time, and I wasn't confident I could provide Ella Rae with adequate nutrition as a vegan. I went back to the drawing board. I had heard rumblings about the Paleo diet, and after reading books and doing research, we decided to make the switch. We went from a completely vegetarian diet to a Paleo diet *overnight*. I hadn't had meat in four years, so it was a pretty rough transition. I had gotten to the point that the mere thought of meat was disgusting to me, so pivoting to thirty days of a meat-focused diet was a challenge!

But I felt the benefits of the switch almost immediately. Chaz and I had more energy, we lost weight, and our skin cleared up. As vegetarians, we'd been legume and grain heavy—two foods my body doesn't tolerate very well. (This is something I wish I'd known much earlier!) When we switched to a Paleo diet, I had zero digestive issues. They were completely gone!

I was so empowered by this new lifestyle and how great we felt that just a month later, I started my blog, Olive You Whole, and started creating recipes to help other people who were on a similar journey. Each person and each family will have their own unique needs and preferences, but the bottom line is the same: What are you eating? Why are you eating it? And is it the best fit for what your body needs? If we don't make intentional choices about the food we consume, we'll end up eating things by default—whatever is in the snack cabinet or the drive-through lane—instead of eating foods that truly fuel our bodies.

What Makes Something a Healthy Food

When you think about the intricate ways God created our bodies, it's really quite remarkable. Without having to consciously think about it, our hearts pump blood to every part of our body, our lungs breathe air, the synapses in our brains fire so we can think and move and communicate, and food is transformed into energy by a series of complex digestive processes. When you consider what a finely tuned machine we've been entrusted with, it's clear that we'd be wise to take good care of it.

You would never think about pouring purple Kool-Aid into your car and hoping it takes you up a mountain pass. Similarly, our bodies were made to be fueled by specific foods. (Spoiler alert: it's not Twinkies.) Food can—and should—be our ally! It is quite literally our fuel; it gives us energy to walk and run and jump and play and climb and kayak and parent and work and serve and do #allthethings.

One of the biggest reasons to be intentional about what you eat is so you can feel your best. I often hear from people who start prioritizing real, whole foods, "I had no idea I could feel this good!" Just because everyone around you eats certain foods, that doesn't mean it's healthy or good for you.

In our household, we try not to have black-and-white lists of "healthy" and "unhealthy" foods. Instead, we talk about "all the time" foods and "sometimes" foods. I think eating any one way 100 percent of the time is not only unrealistic but also harmful mentally. In fact, a legalistic, inflexible diet can make you up to five times more likely to develop an eating disorder.[1] In addition, your social life will take a hit if you are unnecessarily strict about what you eat. (I am not referring to diets that must be strict due to a diagnosis or health condition. If you fall into this camp, you still have options! You can invite friends over and cook for them, or you can host a potluck and offer to make the main meal. You can also contact restaurants in advance to see if they can accommodate your dietary restrictions.)

> ## Checklist for "All the Time" Foods
>
> - Does it make you personally feel great?
> - Does it support your metabolism and stable blood-sugar levels?
> - Does it support satiety between meals?
> - Does it contain fiber to support regular bowel movements?
> - Is it high in vitamins, minerals, and nutrients?
> - Does it keep your mood stable?
> - Does it support a full night of sleep?
> - Does it help you maintain energy throughout the day?
> - Does it support balanced hormones?

So what makes something an "all the time" food for our family? For me, these include foods that are nearly entirely beneficial and not harmful to our bodies.

All-the-Time Foods

Meat and Seafood

Of all the food groups, meat may be the most controversial. We've been sold a lie that meat is at the heart of the climate-change crisis and that if you truly care for the planet, you'll go vegan. As a former near-vegan myself, I am thrilled to tell you that's a bunch of bologna! (Pun intended, and more on processed meat in a minute!) Our family is passionate about eating quality meat for these reasons: it's saving the planet (no, really!),[2] our bodies were designed to eat meat, and it's the most nutrient-dense food on the planet.

Here's the catch, though: all meat is not created equal. Of all the food categories we'll talk about in this chapter, I believe meat is *the* most important food to prioritize in terms of getting the highest quality you can.

Because here's where I do agree with those who advocate against meat consumption: factory-farmed meat is atrocious. These setups are otherwise known as concentrated animal feeding organizations, or CAFOs (pronounced KAY-fohs) in the biz. There are a number of problems with factory-farmed meat—for us and for the environment.

First, it is not ethical. As the name suggests, CAFOs can cram millions of animals together in dry, open feedlots or in windowless buildings—obviously not their natural habitats.[3] Second, it is not safe. CAFOs pollute the surrounding air, soil, and water.[4] The overuse of antibiotics kills weak bacteria and leaves harder-to-treat "superbugs" in their place.[5] In addition, factory-farmed meat is harmful to the land and communities near the CAFO. People who live in the surrounding area have been shown to experience higher rates of diseases and cancer, even among children.[6]

Checklist for "Sometimes" Foods

- Is it created to encourage overeating? (Most packaged foods fall into this category!)
- Does it spike blood sugar (for example, sweets and candy)?
- Does it encourage inflammation?
- Does it disrupt the gut and digestion?
- Is it high in calories and low in nutrition?
- Does it give you negative symptoms (such as migraines, brain fog, hives, trouble sleeping)?
- Does it cause a crash in your energy level?
- Is it addictive (for example, sugar-laden foods)?
- Does it cause future food cravings?

When it comes to all the different foods you could be eating, it can be hard to cut through all the noise to figure out what foods will work best for your body. I'd like to take you through the major food groups and explain what the latest science tells us about the pros and cons in each category. My hope is that by the end of this chapter, you'll be able to find foods that bring you joy, fill your belly and your soul, and bring you vitality and longevity.

Finally, the meat is significantly less nutritious than pasture-raised, regenerative-agriculture meat. Believe it or not, cows in CAFOs are often knowingly fed candy—yes, *candy*. You are what you eat; you also are what you eat *eats*.

I agree that *that* kind of meat is not good. But what about *good* meat? The argument

> **You are what you eat; you also are what you eat *eats*.**

"This type of meat is bad, so all meat is bad and no one should eat meat" is like saying, "The water in Flint, Michigan, is terrible, so all water is terrible and no one should drink water." The issue is not meat or no meat; it's about the quality.

I believe down to my bone marrow that we should eat meat. When animals are raised using regenerative agriculture practices, this not only provides a wonderful food source for us but also improves the health of the earth.

So what does regenerative agriculture mean? It means that farmers take depleted dirt and transform it into a luscious prairie using practices involving ruminant animals (such as cattle, bison, sheep, elk, goat, and deer). What many people don't realize is that transformation—from dirt to soil—actually captures carbon, which helps reduce greenhouse gases. (I know, right?)[7]

I've had the honor of visiting my friends' farm at Roam Ranch (the makers of Force of Nature meats, which you may be able to find in your grocery store!). They did exactly this with their acres of land in Fredericksburg, Texas. When raised and treated the way nature intended, animals can be part of healing our planet.

Another reason to eat meat is simple: because our bodies were made to. Scientists believe that our ancestors' development of fire and ability to cook and eat meat helped their brains grow, which led to increased skills, such as language development.[8]

Meat and seafood are some of the most nutrient-dense foods on the planet. Let's take a look at grass-fed beef liver (often called "nature's multivitamin"). Not only is it high in protein, like other cuts of beef, but

What to Look for When Shopping for Meat and Seafood

Go straight to the source. The ideal option is to buy directly from a local farmer (if you can, find pasture-raised, organic meat near you, even if it's not certified). The farmers make more money, and you're getting local, farmer-direct meat. The same is true if you're lucky enough to live near a coast and can get fresh, wild fish. The next best option, if you don't have local options near you, is to look for organic, pasture-raised, regeneratively raised meats. You want the "100 percent grass fed" label, meaning the cow was fed only grass, never grain. It's true that these meats are more expensive than conventional meat. Even if you can't afford these types of meat, I still believe eating meat is critical for adequate protein intake and a well-balanced diet.

For fish, there are some labels that don't have certification or oversight, such as "all natural," "sustainably caught," "sustainably harvested," "responsibly farmed," or "responsibly caught."[9] The USDA, which handles the organic label, doesn't have standards set for seafood, so if you see seafood marked "organic," that means it's not from the United States. One of the best labels to look for is from the Marine Stewardship Council, called the "certified sustainable seafood" label. This label ensures that you are supporting sustainably managed fisheries that work to maintain healthy fish populations and their ecosystems.[10] Fish can be wild, wild caught, or farmed. Wild fish aren't manipulated by humans in any way prior to being caught. Wild-caught fish are incubated in hatcheries, then released in streams or rivers. These options are preferable to farmed fish, which aren't raised in the wild and can be damaging to local ecosystems.[11]

When it comes to poultry, don't be fooled by labels like "cage free," which just means the chickens don't live in cages. This doesn't guarantee that the birds have access to outdoor space. They can still be packed in a barn with limited space to move around. "Free range" sounds great, but in reality, the birds often have access to as little as two square feet each. They may have just a tiny door to get outside, which they may or may not use. When shopping for poultry, I recommend looking for the "pasture raised" label. This means the chickens are raised in a way that's consistent with the way they naturally live and behave: in a pasture, with the ability to roam around, scratch, and peck (which also improves the soil).[12]

it's also high in heme iron, nucleic acids, B vitamins, carotenoids, and liver enzymes (which help your own liver function). It is packed with other essential vitamins (such as A, C, D, K, and folate) and essential minerals (such as magnesium, phosphorus, zinc, copper, manganese, and selenium).

Some meats you might enjoy include beef, bison, lamb, pork, chicken, turkey, and duck. If you know someone who hunts, you might

Why Buy Organic?

One of the biggest reasons to buy organic is to minimize your exposure to glyphosate, an herbicide that doubles the risk of non-Hodgkin's lymphoma and increases the risk of liver dysfunction.[13] Organic food doesn't allow for the use of glyphosate. Eating organic isn't just healthier for you; it's also healthier for the planet.

If eating organic is beyond your budget, try to prioritize buying organic from the Environmental Working Group's list of "Dirty Dozen." These are the twelve crops with the highest concentration of glyphosate. The 2023 Dirty Dozen list includes strawberries, spinach, kale, collard, mustard greens, peaches, pears, nectarines, apples, grapes, bell peppers, hot peppers, cherries, blueberries, and green beans.[14] Foods found in the "Clean 15" are the safest options to buy conventionally. The 2023 Clean 15 list includes avocados, sweet corn, pineapples, onions, papayas, sweet peas (frozen), asparagus, honeydew melons, kiwis, cabbage, mushrooms, mangoes, sweet potatoes, watermelons, and carrots.[15]

also try venison, elk, quail, and wild boar.

Seafood is packed with nutrients too. It's high in protein, omega-3 fatty acids, calcium, vitamin A, vitamin E, B vitamins, and minerals such as iron, magnesium, manganese, copper, selenium, and zinc.[16] Prioritize smaller fish and shellfish such as anchovies, cod, herring, oysters, salmon, sardines, shrimp, sole, tilapia, and trout, as they are less likely to contain large amounts of mercury than larger fish.

Vegetables

Vegetables are an essential part of any healthy eating plan. They are packed with micronutrients and phytonutrients that are fantastic for our bodies. Phytonutrients are found only in plants, and they protect us from just about every major disease you can think of. Vegetables also contain lots of fiber, vitamins, and minerals. Fiber keeps food moving through our systems (think about your grandparents drinking Metamucil . . .). Most Americans don't get nearly enough fiber, and the best place to get it is from vegetables.

So go ahead—load up your plate with mostly vegetables at every meal—three-fourths of your plate is ideal! Try to eat more than just America's favorite: the potato. The more unusual the vegetable and the deeper in color, the better for you! (Think heirlooms or varieties you rarely see in your grocery store. They're less likely to be genetically altered and mass produced like the more popular vegetables.) Try to eat a wide variety of vegetables, including leafy greens (kale, romaine, spinach, lettuce), cruciferous vegetables (broccoli, cauliflower, brussels sprouts, cabbage), root vegetables (beets, carrots, parsnips, potatoes, sweet potatoes, turnips), fruits that we call vegetables (cucumbers, pumpkin, squash, zucchini), alliums (onions, garlic, shallots), and edible plant stems (celery, asparagus).

Fruits

Fruits have many of the same benefits as vegetables: they contain vitamins, minerals, phytonutrients, fiber, and carbohydrates. Our bodies are trained to like sweet things, and fruits are great . . . in moderation. Think of fruit as a fun side to your meal, but don't let it take over your plate! You don't want fruits to push aside vegetables, which are more nutrient dense, contain higher fiber, are lower in calories, and have a lower sugar content.

Eating different foods and rotating foods is good for you—it ensures that your body doesn't start attacking one food molecule because you eat it all the time. Be sure to eat lots of different types of fruits: citruses, berries, melons, apples, pears, stone fruits, tropical fruits, and subtropical fruits.[17] Diversifying the fruits you eat also maximizes the nutrition you're getting. I find that eating in-season fruits is helpful: berries and watermelon in the summer, apples in the fall, and oranges in the winter.

You might be thinking, *But aren't sweet things bad for me? Won't they spike my blood sugar?* The answer is, it depends. There's a huge difference between eating one orange and drinking sixteen ounces of orange juice, which will immediately spike your blood sugar. When it comes to fruit and blood sugar, eating is better than drinking. In addition, it's all about *how* you eat something. If you're concerned about insulin

Caveats for Vegetables

- Corn is a grain, not a vegetable.
- Green beans and peas are legumes, not vegetables.
- Some people who struggle with irritable bowel syndrome have a hard time digesting raw vegetables. If you are experiencing GI distress, I encourage you to remove fresh vegetables from your diet. Instead, eat vegetables that have been thoroughly cooked, and start with root vegetables while you're healing your gut.

resistance, choose low glycemic index fruits like fresh apricots, oranges, cherries, blueberries, blackberries, raspberries, strawberries, figs, grapefruit, pears, peaches, and plums. You can also eat fruit along with a protein source and a fat source—this will level out your blood-sugar curve. The bottom line is that, in moderation, fruit is good for you and will not cause metabolic issues.

A Caveat for Fruit

If you have a sugar addiction or if you find you have a hard time giving up sweets, it may be helpful to remove fruit from your diet while you detox from sugar. If you want a candy bar and instead eat four dates, your brain is still connecting the addiction with the reward. That means it's time for a break!

Fats and Oils

Starting in the 1950s, scientists proposed that there was a correlation between saturated fats and heart disease, even though there was no clear evidence that a low-fat diet prevented heart disease or promoted weight loss. Nevertheless, by the 1980s, eating low fat was promoted by physicians, the federal government, the food industry, and the popular health media. Ironically, in the same time period that the low-fat approach became accepted as the gold standard for health, Americans on the whole were getting fatter, leading to what many called an "obesity epidemic."[18]

It may be hard to separate the idea of fat on our bodies (especially the fat we don't want) from the fat we eat. But fat is really important to our bodies. Did you know the brain is made up of nearly 60 percent fat?[19] Our bodies need fat for processes such as balancing hormones, creating healthy nerve function, protecting vital organs, and digesting fat-soluble vitamins.

Food is ultimately fuel, and fat is a great source of fuel! Why? It keeps you full for much longer than, say, carbohydrates. If you're trying to lose weight and your body is constantly burning the carbohydrates you're feeding it for energy, it never needs to access your stored body fat for energy, which means you're not losing fat. When your body has access to fat as fuel, it's able to burn the stored fat on your body.

MONOUNSATURATED FATS

Monounsaturated fats are found in both plant and animal sources, and are usually liquid at room temperature. These types of fat are great for you, and including MUFAs in your diet can decrease unhealthy LDL cholesterol, increase "good" HDL cholesterol, lower blood pressure, reduce the risk of certain cancers, and improve insulin sensitivity.[20]

- Olives and olive oil
- Avocados and avocado oil
- Some nuts, nut butters, and nut oils (such as almonds, hazelnuts, and pecans)
- Some seeds (such as pumpkin seeds and sesame seeds)

SATURATED FATS

Saturated fats are found mainly in animal products and are typically solid at room temperature. While it was once believed that high consumption of saturated fats led to cardiovascular problems, this idea is not supported by current evidence. In fact, the two fats in our blood that cause heart attacks (palmitic acid and stearic acid) do not come from eating fats but from eating sugar and carbs.[21]

- Animal fats such as clarified butter (ghee), duck fat, tallow (beef fat), schmaltz (chicken fat), goat fat, lard (pig fat)
- Coconut oil and other coconut products
- Cream, butter, and cheese
- Palm oil and palm kernel oil (prioritize RSPO certified to decrease deforestation)

POLYUNSATURATED FATS

Omega-3s are a beneficial polyunsaturated fat that lowers your "bad" triglycerides. (Higher triglycerides increase your risk of heart disease and stroke.) Omega-3s also benefit heart health by potentially raising "good" cholesterol HDL and lowering blood pressure. In addition to improving heart health, these fats can lower your risk of developing some cancers,

Alzheimer's disease, dementia, and age-related macular degeneration.[22] It's ideal to get omega-3s from whole food sources, but I also take an omega-3 supplement. You can get healthy omega-3s from the following foods:

- Fatty fish
- Seafood
- Eggs
- Grass-fed meat
- Flaxseed
- Algae
- Walnuts

Omega-6s also play a crucial role in brain function, skin and hair growth, bone health, metabolism regulation, and reproductive health. While omega-6s are technically essential, it's all about a healthy balance between omega-3 and omega-6 fatty acids. You don't need to go out of your way to get omega-6s, as the standard American diet has fourteen to twenty-five times more omega-6 than omega-3 fatty acids, mainly through harmful seed oils. The intake of too many omega-6 fatty acids promotes inflammation in the body.[23]

Fat and Oil Quality

It's important to take a couple of things into consideration when buying fats and oils. First, oils can go rancid quickly, so be sure your oil doesn't smell bitter before using it. Additionally, olive oil and avocado oil can be counterfeit! Researchers at the University of California Davis found that 70 percent of the avocado oils they studied were either rancid or mixed with other oils, usually sunflower or safflower (both of which are harmful seed oils).[24] Be sure you're buying extra virgin olive oil and virgin avocado oil. I buy Chosen Foods or Primal Kitchen avocado oil. For saturated fats, aim for organic, pasture-raised, grass-fed butter, tallow, and lard. This is especially important when buying animal-based fats because toxins are stored in the fat.

Eggs

For decades, the government's recommendation was to skip the egg yolk. The theory was that dietary cholesterol caused heart attacks. The US *Scientific Report of the 2015 Dietary Guidelines Advisory Committee* found "no appreciable relationship" between dietary cholesterol and heart disease.[25] Now we know the egg yolk is the most nutritious part of the egg—don't skip it! The yolk contains necessary minerals (such as calcium, zinc, and phosphorous), vitamins (A, D, E, K, and B complex), antioxidants (such as glutathione), and anti-inflammatory omega-3s.[26] As with chicken, look for organic, pasture-raised eggs.

Dairy

Of all the food groups, dairy may be the most confusing. First, we've been hearing misleading messages about dairy for decades. In 2023, dairy lobbies in the United States spent more than $7.5 million on their lobbying efforts—in just one year![27]

The other reason we hear mixed messages about dairy, even within the health and wellness community, is because there's a huge difference between traditional pasteurized, homogenized dairy and raw dairy.

Raw milk contains more than 2,500 proteins, including the enzyme lactase; 400 fatty acids; bioavailable calcium; fat-soluble vitamins such as vitamins A, D, E, and K2; vitamin C; all the B vitamins, including folate (B9) and B12; minerals such as calcium, phosphorus, magnesium, and zinc; and trace minerals such as selenium. It truly is a nearly perfect food, packed with nutrition!

Traditional milk, on the other hand, is legally required to be both pasteurized (to kill harmful bacteria present) and homogenized.[28] Unfortunately, this heating process also kills the naturally occurring enzymes in milk. The more than 2,500 different proteins in milk become denatured during the pasteurization process, including anti-bacterial enzymes and antibodies that help our immune systems.[29]

What are enzymes? Enzymes are proteins that speed up metabolism and other chemical reactions in our bodies.[30] The enzyme alkaline phosphatase is an anti-inflammatory enzyme found in raw milk. Guess what else is an enzyme? Yep, lactase. Lactase is the enzyme that breaks down the lactose found in milk, but lactase is killed in the pasteurization process. This is one of the reasons traditional dairy is harder to digest than raw dairy.

When milk goes through the homogenization process, the fat globules in milk are broken down into extremely small particles and then distributed uniformly throughout.[31] More than 400 fatty acids are destroyed during the homogenization process. Raw dairy, on the other hand, keeps the beneficial properties of the cream. One of these benefits is the Wulzen factor, also called the "anti-stiffness factor," which helps with arthritis because of its anti-inflammatory properties.[32]

When I was trying to get to the root of my gut issues, dairy was one of the first culprits I addressed. I discovered that, along with thirty to fifty million other Americans, I am lactose intolerant.[33] Without the beneficial components of raw milk, traditional milk can have a number of downsides. Consuming traditional milk products can cause inflammatory conditions such as digestive distress, acne, eczema, and allergic reactions. If you have any of these symptoms, try switching to raw milk or removing dairy from your diet altogether for a period of time. When you reintroduce dairy again, eat it once and monitor your body's reactions for a few days.

If you can't tolerate traditional milk, the good news is that your body may be able to handle raw milk or raw milk products such as cream, yogurt, kefir, or cheese. If you can't tolerate those either, try goat products or sheep products. There are some cheeses that can be made with raw milk because of the aging and curing process, which takes place for at least sixty days. These cheeses are available even in states where you can't find raw milk: Asiago, blue cheese, Brie, cotija, feta, fontina, Gruyère, Manchego, Parmigiano-Reggiano (Parmesan cheese), Roquefort, and pecorino.

Where to Find Raw Milk

Raw milk isn't fully legalized in all states because of the risk of foodborne bacteria outbreaks. While the lack of pasteurization is a risk, the important thing is to find a farm you can trust. Tour their facilities and find out if they've ever had any complaints or outbreaks. For perspective, since the Centers for Disease Control (CDC) started tracking foodborne E. coli outbreaks in 2006, seventeen out of forty-nine cases were from leafy greens or sprouts and only two were from dairy products.[34]

All states do allow for the sale of raw milk, but access depends on the state. In some states you can get raw milk through retail outlets, in some states the milk is labeled "for pet consumption only," in some states you have to purchase the milk on the farm itself, and in other states you have to join a cow share. You can look online to find raw milk in your area.

Nuts and Seeds

Nuts are the seeds of fruits, typically contained in a hard shell. Nuts and seeds are healthy sources of protein, fat, fiber, antioxidants, vitamins, minerals, and micronutrients. I love nuts because they don't spike your blood sugar—a major win. They've also been linked with weight loss (especially the loss of harmful visceral belly fat), positive arterial health, lower blood pressure, reduced risk of heart disease and cancer, and prevention of type 2 diabetes. They may even keep you alive longer![35]

There are so many options when it comes to nuts and seeds. I love nuts that are higher in saturated fats, such as Brazil nuts (these are also naturally high in selenium, which is great for thyroid health), cashews, and macadamia nuts. Nuts and seeds that are high in monounsaturated fatty acids include almonds, pistachios, pecans, and hazelnuts, plus pumpkin and sesame seeds. Walnuts, pine nuts, and chia seeds are highest in polyunsaturated fatty acids, some of which are the great kind, omega-3s.

If you like nut milk, be sure to get a brand with the fewest number of ingredients possible—ideally just nuts and water (I like the Malk brand). Avoid nut milk with seed oils, added sugar, and other gums and thickeners, and buy organic, if you can.

Legumes

Legumes (or pulses) include all types of beans, peas, lentils, and peanuts. While there are thousands of species of legumes, some common examples include adzuki beans, black beans, black-eyed peas, cannellini beans, chickpeas, cranberry beans, fava beans, great northern beans, green beans, kidney beans, lentils and split lentils, lima beans, mung beans, navy beans, peanuts, peas and split peas, pinto beans, sugar snap peas, snow peas, and soybeans.

Legumes contain phytates, or antinutrients, that grab hold of minerals like calcium, iron, zinc, and magnesium, making many types of beans indigestible and unable to be absorbed by our bodies. Bacteria ferment these undigested carbohydrates and cause gas and bloating (which you may be all too familiar with!).

A note on soy specifically: according to the Harvard School of Public Health, there is conflicting data on the effects of soy on the body. Some people sing its praises. Others are hesitant to wholeheartedly welcome it into their diet because of concerns about estrogen-mimicking effects.[36] If you tolerate soy well and choose to include it in your diet, there are benefits: it is relatively inexpensive and packed with protein and B vitamins, potassium, and magnesium. However, soy is one of the crops sprayed most heavily with glyphosate, and it is often genetically modified, so choosing organic soy products is especially important.

All that said, legumes have redeeming qualities. They are eaten all around the world because they are high in protein and low in cost. Legumes and beans are rich in plant protein, fiber, B vitamins, iron, folate, calcium, potassium, phosphorus, and zinc. Most beans are also low in fat. Beans and legumes contain antioxidants that help prevent cell damage and fight disease.[37] When it comes to legumes, I recommend doing some experimenting to see how your body tolerates them.

Sometimes Foods

"Sometimes" foods are foods you want to minimize or include in your eating pattern only occasionally. As we've discussed, it's counterproductive to have legalistic rules around certain foods, but you also don't want to make them a daily part of your eating routine.

Sugar

Our bodies were made to crave sweetness. When we taste something sweet, it's meant to signal to our brains that what we're eating is a great, micronutrient-dense source of energy—in other words, fruit. But in the era of processed food, sweetness no longer means just fruit; it's also food that gives the high of sugar but doesn't provide the fiber and nutrients of fruit.

Food creators know that sugar will light up the pleasure, emotion, and reward centers of the brain. The result? Sugar cravings. We eat a bite of something, and we immediately want more.

Sugar can promote leptin and insulin resistance, cause leaky gut, and lead to nonalcoholic fatty liver disease, among other complications.[38] Studies show that ingesting too much sugar significantly increases the risk of dying from cardiovascular disease.[39]

If sugar isn't a healthy option for our bodies, what about artificial sweeteners? Unfortunately, these sweeteners are no better for you than sugar. An early artificial sweetener called cyclamate was banned by the FDA in 1970 due to severe carcinogenic risks found in animal trials.[40] More long-term studies are needed, but scientists believe there's a relationship between the consumption of artificial sweeteners and certain cancers, chronic fatigue syndrome, Parkinson's disease, Alzheimer's disease, multiple sclerosis, autism, and lupus.[41] Additionally, the sweetness in artificial sweeteners can trigger an unnecessary insulin release and can negatively impact the makeup of the gut microbiome, which can lead to insulin resistance.[42] There's enough doubt about the safety of artificial sweeteners that my take is, why risk it?

When our family wants something sweet, we tend to use natural alternatives to sugar like honey, maple syrup, and coconut sugar. These are lower on the glycemic index than sugar and offer enzymes, vitamins, minerals, and antioxidants that aren't present in traditional sugar.[43] As with anything, they should be used in moderation!

Seed Oils

Vegetable oil sounds healthy, like it's made from good-for-you vegetables, but it's almost always canola and soy oil. Soy (mainly in the form of oil) accounts for up to 10 percent of Americans' calories.[44] Our intake of soy increased one-thousand-fold between 1909 and 1999.[45]

These oils are high in polyunsaturated fats (PUFAs) and omega-6s, and they promote systemic inflammation. Inflammation, in turn, contributes to obesity, insulin resistance, type 2 diabetes, cancer, and many other health concerns.[46] You may not think you consume much seed oil, but it's an ingredient in all kinds of foods.

Seed Oils to Avoid

- Canola (rapeseed) oil
- Corn oil
- Cottonseed oil
- Grape-seed oil
- Peanut oil
- Rice bran oil
- Safflower oil
- Soybean oil
- Sunflower oil

Trans Fats

Most trans fats are partially hydrogenated oils that should stay off your plate as much as possible. They have been shown to cause heart attacks. It's easier to avoid these fats now because the FDA banned them entirely in 2015.[47]

Grains

This might surprise you, but we don't need to eat any grains at all! Even though you can thrive without them, grains are by far the number-one source of calories for Americans, coming in at 581 calories from grains per person, per day.[48] When eaten in their highly processed form of white flour, grains are essentially sugar, and your body processes them as if they are (and responds with a huge insulin surge). Eating grains has been linked to obesity, heart disease, type 2 diabetes, dementia, and even cancer.[49]

Gluten is a protein found in grains such as wheat, barley, rye, and triticale. Recent research indicates that it's not just those with celiac disease or non-celiac gluten sensitivity who should avoid gluten. Gluten causes everyone's gut lining to become compromised, creating what's known as leaky gut syndrome and allowing particles into the bloodstream that shouldn't be there.[50] While Ella Rae, Owen, and I can't tolerate gluten, I do think it's important to make the distinction that not all grains, even the gluten-containing ones, are created equal. The grains we're eating today are substantially different from what our great-grandparents ate. They've been altered through cross-breeding and are often monocrops, which destroy the environment. (A monocrop is when the same crop is grown in a field over and over again.) On top of that, traditional (non-organic) grains are heavily sprayed with glyphosate, a known toxin. Some forms of gluten-containing grains are more easily tolerated, like the ancient grains Kamut and einkorn, especially in the form of sourdough.

If you're going to eat grains, here's what I recommend: avoid gluten as much as possible, eat organic

Weird Grains to Try

- Black (purple), brown, red, or wild rice
- Amaranth
- Millet
- Quinoa
- Sorghum
- Teff
- Whole kernel, on-the-cob, organic corn

grains and whole grains (not their refined flours), eat "weird grains," and make grains an infrequent part of your eating habits.

If you struggle with inflammation, have an autoimmune disease, are struggling with a metabolic disease, have high blood sugar or diabetes, are trying to lose weight, or have digestive issues, I would recommend avoiding grains altogether.

The Extras

Drinks

When sugar is in liquid form, like in drinks, it spikes blood sugar much faster and more drastically than when you eat it. For example, it's much better to eat an orange than to drink orange juice. For this reason, my "all the time" options for drinks include filtered water (more on hydration in chapter 4), fermented liquids like kefir and kombucha, teas (herbal, green, and white), and fresh cold-pressed juices (try to shoot for more veggies than fruits in these).

Handling Cravings

When you're switching to a new lower-sugar diet, you might get hit with cravings. What I've found is that when I get a craving for something sweet, it's usually a cue that I'm hungry. When a craving hits, I try to have a snack that's high in protein and fat, and 95 percent of the time my craving goes away! If the craving persists, I try to find a healthier alternative to whatever I'm craving—maybe fruit or dark chocolate.

I think every human being, myself included, has used eating as a coping strategy. When you have a craving, take a moment to pause and consider why. Maybe it truly is hunger, or maybe you just got a stress-evoking email from your boss, you're feeling sad about a recent breakup, or you're simply bored. Part of the journey toward a healthier lifestyle is noticing these triggers and replacing negative coping strategies with positive ones. I've found that when it comes to cravings, I usually want something that feels fun in the moment. And while a midday cocktail might sound fun, replacing it with sparkling water and a lime fulfills the same desire.

If you're going to drink coffee, be sure it is an organic, mold-free brand like Kion, and never drink it on an empty stomach. Your body needs energy when you wake up in the morning. When you drink coffee on an empty stomach, instead of getting energy from the food you eat, your body will instead spike your cortisol (a stress hormone) to raise your blood sugar.

Mindfulness around Eating

When you're learning to eat in a new way, it's important to practice mindfulness, which simply means being present and aware of the food you're eating, starting with making it all the way through to enjoying it. In contrast to our grab-and-go society, mindful eating helps you be intentional about slowing down and savoring your food. This helps you notice what you're eating and remember how food makes you feel. Keeping a food journal can be helpful in this process. Some foods disrupt your ability to know when you're full. Eventually, you'll learn to tune in to, understand, and honor your hunger cues. Ideally, you will eat when you're hungry and stop when you're full.

You will also start to notice which foods keep you satiated longer (likely protein and fat). Another component of mindful eating is stopping other activities during mealtimes. Did you know that if you're in a stressed state, your body doesn't digest food as well? When you sit down to fully focus on a meal, it helps your body get into a parasympathetic "rest and digest" state. Fun fact: taking a moment to pray before a meal is good for both your spiritual life and your health, because it helps you pause and get calm before diving in. Another aid in digestion is to fully chew your food. It might sound like a small thing, but breaking your food down into digestible pieces is a critical part of knowing when you're full. As a nutritionist once told me, "Chew your liquids and drink your solids!"

If you opt to drink alcohol, drink infrequently and in moderate amounts, which is defined as no more than one drink per day for women and two drinks per day for men (a drink is defined as twelve ounces of beer, five ounces of wine, or one and a half ounces of hard liquor (on its own or in a cocktail). One way to keep drinking in check is to set boundaries, such as drinking only at the Sabbath dinner or only on special occasions. If you decide to drink alcohol, I recommend drinking in community and choosing alcohols that are made without harmful pesticides and have lower levels of alcohol, sugar, and sulfites. A good wine option that you can easily get is Dry Farm Wines.

Herbs, Spices, and Salts

Herbs are some of the most nutritionally dense foods on the planet. For this reason, I grow and buy fresh herbs as often as possible, and they are staples in nearly all our meals. Try to buy organic herbs and spices, and avoid flavoring packets that contain additives, preservatives, sugar, and standard table salt. Aim for a whole-food diet, and avoid extra ingredients like thickeners, emulsifiers, and preservatives.

In recent years, there has been a war on sodium in an attempt to decrease high blood pressure and subsequently heart attacks, strokes, and other health concerns. One study of more than ten thousand people in thirty-two different countries found no correlation between salt intake and hypertension.[51] Just like anything else, the key is balance.

Salt provides an opportunity to get minerals into your diet. Despite its negative reputation, salt is an electrolyte that helps your body function optimally. When you're eating primarily whole, unprocessed foods, salt is a great addition to your diet. And as you can probably guess, quality is everything. You do *not* want to buy processed table salt.

> ### Tips for Making Healthy Food More Affordable
>
> - Eat seasonally (usually the produce on sale is in season)
> - Stock up on shelf-stable or freezable items when they're on sale
> - Buy dried instead of canned beans
> - Buy grains, beans, nuts, and spices in bulk
> - Make your own sauces, condiments, and salad dressings
> - Shop local
> - Buy healthy groceries at a discount at Thrive Market
> - Use apps that pay you to shop (like Ibotta, Fetch, or Checkout 51)
> - Use coupons directly from the grocery stores where you shop, or use apps like SnipSnap, a community-driven app that gathers coupons
> - Try Imperfect Foods or Misfits Market
> - Don't buy beverages (drink water instead)
> - Minimize snack purchases (focus on whole foods instead of chips, crackers, and packaged foods)

Instead, opt for a more nutritionally dense salt such as Himalayan sea salt or Redmond Real Salt—unrefined, natural sea salt that is full of trace minerals. Iodine is added to table salt because Americans don't get much iodine otherwise, and it's an important element for our bodies, especially when it comes to optimal thyroid function. When you switch salts, ensure that you're getting adequate iodine intake through seaweed, fish, shellfish, or supplements.

A Healthy Plate

Now that you know which foods are to be maximized and minimized, how do you craft a healthy plate? Harvard's "Healthy Eating Plate" suggests drinking mainly water and eating moderate amounts of vegetables and healthy proteins, plus some whole grains, fruits, and healthy fats.[52] I also love certified holistic nutritionist Kelly Leveque's "Fab 4" plan, which focuses on stabilizing blood sugar. She suggests that every meal should be made up of clean protein, fat, fiber, and greens. This helps you balance blood sugar fuels, access energy, curb cravings, and shed excess pounds.[53] I try to eat around four ounces of an animal-based protein per meal, which ensures I'm getting twenty to thirty grams of protein three times a day. Then I fill my plate with mostly vegetables and small sources of fats, legumes, fruit, and the occasional grain.

The 80/20 Rule

If this clean way of eating feels overwhelming to you, don't be scared! Not many people eat this way 100 percent of the time. Instead, aim to eat this way 80 percent of the time. The other 20 percent is up to you and depends on what you deem worth it. My 20 percent may be filled with chocolate cake and Mexican food. Yours may be sweet tea and Lay's potato chips. This kind of intentional eating doesn't have to dominate your life. Having fun with friends and food is an important part of life too.

Food Challenge

Beginner challenge: Replace all your beverages with filtered water, sparkling water, and herbal tea. Hydration is a foundation for health, and we often don't realize how little water we're drinking when we're consuming sodas and coffee.

Intermediate challenge: For one month, choose one food group from the "sometimes foods" list to minimize: sugar, seed oils, or grains (or something else of your choice). Monitor your progress throughout the month, and you might be surprised by how much better you feel!

Advanced challenge: For one month, eat only foods from the "all the time" list: meats and seafood, vegetables, fruits, healthy fats and oils, nuts and seeds, raw dairy, and legumes (if well tolerated). Take notes about how you feel as the month goes on. For clean-eating recipes, check out my cookbook *Prep, Cook, Freeze* and the recipes at my website, oliveyouwhole.com.

CHAPTER 3

MOVE HARD, SLEEP HARD

Eating alone will not keep a man well; he must also take exercise.

HIPPOCRATES

You might be wondering why this chapter pairs two seemingly opposite topics: exercise and sleep. After all, one is about moving your body and the other is about staying in roughly one position. But here's the thing: if you want to sleep hard, you have to move hard too! Okay, not *hard*, as we'll soon discuss, but movement goes hand in hand with great sleep. They're not opposites; they're more like complements—they go together like peanut butter and jelly (or tea and crumpets, if you prefer!).

Both science and the Bible have a lot to say about the connection between movement and rest. According to Charlene Gamaldo, medical director of Johns Hopkins Center for Sleep, "We have solid evidence that exercise does, in fact, help you fall asleep more quickly and improves sleep quality."[1]

The Bible also talks about moving our bodies and resting. In

1 Corinthians 9:25-27, Paul describes the discipline of physical training and how it relates to our spiritual lives: "All athletes are disciplined in
their training. They do it to win a prize that will fade away, but we do it
for an eternal prize. So I run with purpose in every step. . . . I discipline
my body like an athlete, training it to do what it should" (NLT). But
God also makes it clear that our bodies need rest—and that he delights
in giving us that rest: "In peace I will lie down and sleep, for you alone,
O Lord, will keep me safe" (Psalm 4:8, NLT).

Exercise Trends

Until as recently as the 1920s, having a bigger, fatter body was a sign of
wealth. It meant you could afford plenty of food and other people to do
manual labor for you.

It wasn't until the early 1930s that women's fitness started gaining
popularity. The Women's League of Health and Beauty (now Flexercise)
was founded in 1930 in England. Prunella Stack, sometimes called "the
foremother of women's fitness," grew the WLHB to a worldwide membership of 170,000 women by 1938, encouraging women to embrace
Pilates, aerobics, dance exercise, and yoga.[2]

The 1940s saw a stretching trend, and Hula-Hooping as a form of
exercise became popular in the 1950s (can we bring this one back?). The
vibrating belt came into fashion in the 1960s (unsurprisingly, this didn't
work to "shake the fat away" and didn't last long). The 1970s brought
us Jazzercise (which introduced us to the craze of dancing as a workout
and is still around today).

It wasn't until the 1980s that there was a consensus in the US that
everyone should be doing some kind of exercise.[3] The decade was
marked by the aerobics craze, complete with brightly colored Jane
Fonda–inspired leotards.

The 1990s lauded Suzanne Somers's ThighMaster, the 2000s gave
rise to Zumba (still alive and well!), and the 2010s were dominated by
two very different exercises: CrossFit and yoga.[4]

In the 2020s, there seems to be a turn toward specific gym-based fitness programs such as Orangetheory and F45. The global pandemic also led to a surge in at-home workouts, with Peloton increasing in popularity, along with other online workout platforms.

Despite the wide array of exercise options available to us, we as a culture are increasingly sedentary. The need for movement aside from work is a relatively new phenomenon. The very idea of "working out" is only about a hundred years old. In previous generations, people didn't have a frame of reference for hitting the gym. Their daily activities—hunting, gathering, farming, or doing manual labor—were inherently active pursuits. Our bodies are wired toward inactivity so we can save our energy for the tasks required for survival.[5] Unfortunately, this "be lazy" messaging no longer serves us when we're not, in fact, going to hunt antelope for three days in a row . . .

Until the industrial revolution, most work was manual labor. In the nineteenth and twentieth centuries, we started to rely more on machinery, mechanization, and automation than manual labor. Then, in the 1990s and early 2000s, the internet took a lot of jobs online. In recent history, especially following 2020, many workers shifted to online work, with a number of positions going fully remote. Jobs dependent on intense strength and labor continue to decrease.

According to the US Bureau of Labor Statistics, 29 percent of all jobs in America are sedentary, 33 percent require light physical work, 29 percent require medium work, 8 percent require heavy work, and one percent require very heavy work.[6] In other words, a lot of us don't move much for our jobs. I can work from just about anywhere with Wi-Fi and my laptop (someone invite me to Bali, please!). I got so tired of sitting so much for my work that I recently upgraded to a standing desk with a treadmill underneath. It's easy for many of us to work for hours at a time without moving at all. This shift away from manual labor means that a lot of us have to be intentional about moving our bodies—and we need to look outside our jobs to make it happen.

Move Over, Exercise

As our assumptions about work have changed, the way we think about movement has shifted too. Instead of generally moving our bodies throughout the day, we now think of exercise as a very specific type of movement. We think it means going to a gym, weight lifting, running on a treadmill, or ellipticaling. (Can that be a verb? I just made it one!) I think this narrow view of exercise has been extremely harmful for us. It means that for everyone except the select few who adore going to a gym, all the joy has been sucked out of the idea of moving our bodies.

Another consequence of this shift is the idea that we should exercise out of guilt or as a type of punishment for eating certain foods that have been deemed bad. It's as if we've come up with some sort of checks and balances for what we eat and how we should move. Eat a donut? That's thirty minutes on the treadmill. As we discussed in chapter 2, having a legalistic attitude about food is not helpful. In fact, this kind of mentality often has the opposite effect—the more we deny ourselves and punish ourselves, the less likely we are to stick with a lifestyle of balanced, healthy habits.

> The most important factor when it comes to moving your body isn't about muscle mass, high intensity, rigor, or variability. It's *joy.*

If you feel like you have limited options for exercise and you abhor all of them, you'll never move your body! This is not an attainable, long-term goal. If you struggle to exercise consistently, I'd like to propose a new way to think about moving your body. It's time to move away from the traditional ideas about exercise and toward a more encompassing perspective geared toward movement in many different forms.

The most important factor when it comes to moving your body isn't about muscle mass, high intensity, rigor, or variability. It's *joy.* Why? Because what's equally important to the workout itself is longevity. You need to find something you enjoy, because that means you'll do it often and for a long time—maybe even your whole life!

I'm sure you've tried new forms of exercise you hated. Or maybe you attempted one and thought, *There are way too many barriers to keeping up with this activity.* Maybe you had a friend who loved a certain type of movement. It worked for their schedule, their personality, and their fitness goals. My friend Jenny invited me to her F45 class, which she loved because of the quick exercises, frequent rotations, and community vibe. She also went to the 5:30 a.m. class so she could get to work on time. On the one hand, I appreciated that I could be done and home before the kids even got up. But after my week trial, I was kind of over it. And after Jenny moved, I was even less motivated to make it happen.

That's why I recommend trying different activities so you can find something you love doing. And you don't have to choose just one form of movement—it's great to have some variety! So instead of thinking you have to pay for an expensive gym membership or become a weight lifting champion, I encourage you to think outside of the box a bit.

The Centers for Disease Control and Prevention recommends 150 minutes of moderate-intensity physical activity (such as brisk walking), plus two days of muscle-strengthening activity each week. I know that might sound like a lot, but it breaks down to just thirty minutes of movement five times a week, plus some strength training. For the sake of illustration, that's thirty minutes of movement every weekday and no movement on the weekends. You can also do vigorous-intensity aerobic activities such as jogging or running for a shorter time—just seventy-five minutes a week—or a mix of the two.

The CDC also notes that any movement is better than none and that overall we should be shooting for more movement and less sitting. Any amount of moderate-to-vigorous intensity physical activity gives you some benefit.[7]

The Benefits of Movement

There are so many benefits of movement that it's hard to list them all. According to the CDC, "regular physical activity is one of the most important things you can do for your health."[8] It keeps your brain sharp, improves overall brain health, reduces the risk of disease, strengthens muscles and bones, and improves your ability to complete everyday activities.[9] Moving your body also supports the immune system and helps your body detoxify.[10] When you're moving your body, your heart rate increases. This stimulates blood flow to the brain, which in turn provides more oxygen and nutrients. Strengthening your muscles increases the mitochondria in your body, which in turn increases your metabolism.

Exercise is also great for your hormones. It decreases the stress hormones adrenaline and cortisol while increasing your endorphins.[11] Not only does exercise create an anti-inflammatory state in the body, it also guards against chronic, inflammation-associated diseases.[12]

In addition to all these benefits, movement positively affects mental health. Recent studies report some incredible perks of exercise: "Exercise is more beneficial for conditions such as anxiety and depression than standard psychotherapy or medications."[13] According to one study, "physical activity is 1.5 times more effective at reducing mild-to-moderate symptoms of depression, psychological stress, and anxiety than medication or cognitive behavior therapy."[14] In other words, moving your body is great for your body *and* your mind.

Which Types of Movement Are Right for You?

There are different types of movement, and each one provides unique benefits for our bodies. The major categories of movement are cardio, strength training, and stretching.

Cardio

Cardiovascular or aerobic exercise (often shortened to "cardio") has many benefits. Cardio refers to activities that increase the heart rate and respiration level using large muscle groups, often in repetitive or rhythmic ways. This type of movement is important because it challenges your most vital internal network, improving the function and performance of your heart, lungs, and circulatory system.[15]

This kind of movement helps with weight management, increases your stamina and strength, boosts your immune system, and reduces your risk for obesity, heart disease, high blood pressure, type 2 diabetes, metabolic syndrome, stroke, and certain types of cancer. It also helps in managing chronic conditions such as high blood sugar, coronary artery disease, and arthritis. As you age, cardio exercise helps you maintain mobility and protects your mind.[16]

With cardio exercise, you quickly feel its effects. When your body needs more oxygen, your breathing speeds up. Your heart beats faster, increasing the blood flow and oxygen to your muscles. Your body also releases the endorphin dopamine, which is often called the "happy hormone." Endorphins are your body's natural painkillers, and they're what make you feel good after working out. Endorphins can reduce pain, lower stress, improve your mood, and enhance your sense of well-being.[17]

The Benefits of Walking

If you're not sure where to begin when it comes to adding movement to your routine, I'd suggest starting with walking. It's completely free, you don't need any expensive equipment, it is relatively easy to do, and it's great for you! Walking for just thirty minutes a day at a brisk pace is associated with the following benefits:

- Increased cardiovascular (heart) and pulmonary (lung) fitness
- Reduced risk of heart disease and stroke
- Improved management of conditions such as hypertension (high blood pressure), high cholesterol, joint and muscular pain or stiffness, and diabetes
- Stronger bones
- Improved balance
- Increased muscle strength and endurance
- Reduced body fat[18]

Strength Training

Strength training is a kind of exercise that involves using equipment or your own body weight to build muscle mass, endurance, and strength. This may also be referred to as weight lifting, weight training, resistance training, or muscular training. You might think of bodybuilders when you hear these terms, but there are many different ways to go about strength training. You can use heavy weights and low repetitions (or

Ideas to Get Moving

- Walk. (Get creative here! Meet a friend at a coffee shop, and then walk with your coffee! Walk your kiddo to school or walk to the library. Walk your dog. Park far from the store entrance to get some extra steps in.)
- Use a walking treadmill (more of an investment) or a seated, under-desk bike pedal exerciser (more affordable) to get some movement even while you're working!
- Skip the elevator and take the stairs.
- Do free online exercise videos or apps.
- Play with your kids outside (I get some solid movement chasing them around the playground!).
- Do one exercise paired with something you do often (for example, every time you fill up your water, do twenty squats or ten push-ups).
- Do ab exercises (you can do this without equipment or you can use a Pilates ball to enhance stabilization muscles).
- Hike or garden.
- Do rigorous housework, such as vacuuming.
- Swim laps.
- Play water polo.
- Do water aerobics.
- Ride a bicycle (indoor or outdoor).
- Make love (really, it counts!).
- Play sports (such as soccer, basketball, racquetball, tennis, football, volleyball, softball, jujitsu, bowling).
- Take a dance or Zumba class.
- Lift weights.
- Do strength training.
- Do Pilates, yoga, martial arts, tai chi, boxing, kickboxing, CrossFit, high-intensity interval training (HIIT), or resistance training with bands or a TRX system.
- Rebound on a small trampoline.
- Do rigorous yard work.
- Go kayaking.
- Go skiing, snowboarding, or snowshoeing.
- Participate in waterskiing or water sports.
- Go rollerblading (indoor or outdoor) or ice-skating.
- Jump rope or Hula-Hoop.
- Go skateboarding or rock climbing.
- Play Frisbee.
- Walk or run up stairs.
- Play paintball.
- Go paddleboarding.
- Exercise with a buddy (studies show that having a friend join you in your movement of choice evokes the same chemicals in the body as a runner's high).[19]

reps), or you can use light weights and lots of reps. The equipment (or lack thereof) can vary significantly too. You can do body-weight workouts, use free weights (such as dumbbells, barbells, or kettlebells), resistance bands, machines, or suspension equipment (such as TRX systems).

There are many benefits to strength training. It makes you stronger, builds muscle, strengthens your bones, increases your metabolism, and decreases abdominal fat or visceral fat, which is associated with increased risk of chronic diseases, such as heart disease, liver disease, type 2 diabetes, and certain types of cancer. Strength training decreases your risk of falls, lowers your risk of injury, and improves heart health. It helps you maintain a healthy body weight, promotes mobility and flexibility, and boosts your mood.[20]

Stretching

Stretching and balancing activities such as Pilates, yoga, or tai chi are helpful for improving the flexibility of a muscle or muscle group and overall range of motion. Improved flexibility and range of motion have been shown to improve performance in physical activities, decrease risk of injury, help joints move through their full range of motion, increase blood flow to the muscles, improve muscle performance, and improve the execution of daily activities.[21]

While I stand by my philosophy that the best way to stick with moving your body is to find something you enjoy, it's also important to incorporate some variability into your routine. Why? Because each form of movement provides different benefits to our bodies. In order to gain all the benefits, the ideal is to choose something you enjoy from each category.

I tend to base my workouts on how I'm feeling. When I have lots of energy, I'll do a high-intensity workout. When I'm feeling unmotivated, when I'm lacking energy, or when I'm on my cycle, I stick to low-intensity movement (I especially love yoga!).[22] These exercise options are not a "choose one and done" scenario—it's more of a menu to choose from based on your personal situation and how you're feeling.

The Science of Sleep

Just as we need to focus on moving our bodies, we also need to be intentional about resting them. Have you ever thought about the fact that we spend one-third of our lives sleeping? That's the biggest chunk of time we dedicate to doing any single thing!

You may not have given much thought to sleep, but it is foundational for much of what happens when we're awake. In chapter 2 we talked about how food can serve as fuel for our bodies, but sleep gives us the energy we need to live our lives! Getting adequate, restful sleep is absolutely foundational for our overall health and wellness.

While there's a lot that scientists still don't know about sleep, we do know our bodies and minds undergo essential processes while we sleep. During sleep, our memories are consolidated, which helps with emotional regulation.[23] Sleep is also one of the ways our bodies heal, as cells are repaired during sleep. When we sleep, our energy is restored and hormones are released. Nerve cells communicate with one another and reorganize, and accumulated toxic waste byproducts are removed, all of which supports healthy brain function.[24]

Did you know that preventing someone from sleeping is actually a torture tactic? (And all the mamas reading this book called, "Amen"!) After the attacks on the World Trade Center in 2001, the CIA's detention and interrogation program used "enhanced interrogation techniques" that included sleep deprivation, even though the United States has signed the United Nations Convention against Torture and Other Cruel, Inhuman or Degrading Treatment or Punishment.[25] As a result of this sleep deprivation, at least five detainees experienced disturbing hallucinations. Sleep deprivation is considered an especially insidious form of torture, because it "attacks the deep biological functions at the core of a person's mental and physical health."[26]

You may not be detained in a torture situation, but you may be all too familiar with what happens when you don't get enough sleep. What are the first signs of sleep deprivation? According to *Psychology Today*, you experience "unpleasant feelings of fatigue, irritability, and difficulties concentrating. Then come problems with reading and speaking clearly, poor judgment, lower body temperature, and a considerable increase in appetite. If the deprivation continues, the worsening effects include disorientation, visual misperceptions, apathy, severe lethargy, and social withdrawal."[27] Studies show a correlation between inadequate sleep and a wide range of health problems, including hypertension, obesity, and type 2 diabetes. Lack of sleep has also been linked to impaired immune functioning, cardiovascular disease, mood disorders, dementia, and even loneliness.[28]

How Much Sleep Should You Get?

The amount of sleep we need depends on our age. This is why newborn babies come home and you barely find them awake! At this stage, they need up to seventeen hours of sleep a day. As children grow up, their sleep goals decrease slightly every year, with teens having a sleep goal of eight to ten hours (they're still growing!).[29] According to the Sleep Foundation, adults should aim to get seven or more hours of sleep per night.[30]

Are You Getting Enough Sleep?

Ask yourself these questions to determine if you need to get more sleep.

- Do you feel fully rested when you wake up?
- Do you have energy during the day to accomplish your needed tasks?
- Do you have an afternoon slump that is hard to push through?
- Are you at high risk for a disease and would benefit from more sleep?
- Do you have a labor-intensive job or an active lifestyle that requires additional energy?
- Do you depend on caffeine to make it through the day?
- Do you sleep excessively on the weekends or when you're not working?

As with the other suggestions in this book, these guidelines are bio-individual. You may need more or less sleep than your peers do. So how can you find out how much sleep you need? You can try a sleep test! (I recommend trying this on a weekend or a day you don't need to be somewhere the next morning.)

Try to go to sleep around your normal time or a little earlier, if you can fall asleep quickly. Then see how long you sleep without an alarm. (If you have young children, try having your partner or a babysitter watch the kids, since they are a built-in alarm clock!)

How many hours did you sleep? Let's say you slept a glorious nine hours. That means that if you need to wake up at 6 a.m. during the week, try going to bed at 9 p.m. so you can get those full nine hours.

Why Is It Hard to Sleep?

Regardless of the science behind it, we've all felt the implications of a lack of sleep. Whether it's staying up late cramming for a big exam, taking a red-eye flight, working the late shift, or caring for a newborn or someone who is ill, I'm sure you've experienced the effects of inadequate sleep.

The first few months of my son Owen's life, he was the cutest, squishiest, happiest baby during the day. But he would fuss *all night*. I would go into his room and feed him about every forty-five minutes for thirty minutes. You do the math—essentially I wasn't sleeping. And, man, did I feel it! During the day, I was like a zombie.

There are many reasons we don't sleep enough—some of them are a result of factors outside our control and others are a result of choices we make. One of the biggest reasons we don't get enough sleep is because of hustle culture. Unfortunately, it's a socially accepted phenomenon to work hard into the night. We prioritize productivity and work above sleep, thinking we can ignore the

You're Not Welcome in My Bedroom

You might feel like you're missing an appendage when your phone isn't with you, but there are some really good reasons to keep it out of your bedroom.

- If your phone isn't in your bedroom, you can't doomscroll before bed, which has been proven to increase anxiety.[31]
- Social media usage is linked to poor sleep quality.[32]
- Phones cause distraction and stress, especially when we check them first thing in the morning.[33]
- If your face isn't glued to a screen, you're much more likely to have moments of connection with your family before bed. Chaz is faithful about brushing and flossing every night, and that encourages me to brush and floss with him. During our nighttime routine, we often chat about our days—what was hard, what was good. This is a great time to wind down together and connect instead of mindlessly and independently using our phones.

Things That Promote Good Sleep

- Getting adequate movement during the day
- Not drinking caffeine within eight hours of bedtime
- Having a consistent sleep schedule—going to sleep at the same time and waking up at the same time each day
- Minimizing blue light from screens in the evening
- Having a calming nighttime routine
- Reading a book before going to sleep
- Taking a hot bath with Epsom salts in the evening
- Using lavender, cedarwood, or vetiver essential oils (these can be applied topically or used aromatically before going to bed)
- Drinking calming teas and taking supplements (such as melatonin for short-term use to establish a healthy circadian rhythm, jujube seed extract, gamma-aminobutyric acid (GABA), L-theanine, taurine, Glycine, chamomile, lavender, valerian root, ashwagandha, and tulsi teas)
- Taking magnesium (I like Magnesium Breakthrough from BiOptimizers)
- Eating a snack before bed (low blood sugar can cause a cortisol spike, which will wake you up)
- Making your room dark (you can use blackout shades or a sleep mask, or both)
- Minimizing noises (if you don't have control of the noises around you, try using earplugs)
- Regulating your room temperature (sleeping in a room that's overly hot or cold can disrupt your sleep)
- Putting your phone in another room

limitations of being human. We push through and try to make up for it with an extra cup of coffee in the morning.

The work-from-home boom exacerbated this problem, because it further blurred the boundaries between work and home. When you don't go to an office and instead your work is in your home, it can be hard to turn it off, even when your workday is over.

Practicing Good Sleep Hygiene

We need good sleep. We want good sleep. But if you're in the 10 percent of the population worldwide who experience insomnia and other sleep disruptions,[34] sleep may sound like something out of a fairy tale. The good news is that there are practical steps you can take to achieve adequate, restful sleep.

When you think about sleep, you might think about how dark your environment is. What you might not realize is that sunlight actually plays an important role in sleep! Sunlight and moonlight are what set our circadian rhythms. Circadian rhythms are physical, mental, and behavioral changes that follow a twenty-four-hour cycle.[35] Think of your circadian rhythm like your body's clock. This affects your sleep schedule and how your body knows when to fall asleep, but the effects go even deeper than that. Your circadian rhythm also affects hormone release, eating habits, digestion, and your body temperature.

So how exactly does light affect your circadian rhythm? When there is less light coming to your brain from your eyes, it signals to your brain that it must be time to get sleepy, so it starts making melatonin (a hormone that makes you sleepy).[36] In previous generations, without artificial light, people naturally followed the pattern of light outside. They would sleep when it was dark and be awake during daylight hours. But now that we rely on artificial light, especially our blue-light screens, and spend less time outside, our bodies don't experience these natural triggers telling us when to sleep and when to wake up.

There are two action items to note here. The first is the importance of being exposed to natural light as soon as you wake up. If you can take a walk shortly after you wake up or just sit by a bright window, it will help you maintain a healthy circadian rhythm. If you have trouble sleeping, this one habit alone can dramatically improve your sleep!

Second, it's crucial to create a dark environment when it's getting close to bedtime. This is a signal to your body that it's time to start preparing for sleep. My family tries to use only dim, yellow-light lamps in the evening instead of bright lights. You might not think of screens as being a source of light, but the blue lights that come from screens— whether the television, your laptop, or your phone—can incorrectly signal to your brain that it's still daytime. If you have trouble falling asleep or you look at screens during the day, you might benefit from setting a time in the evening when you stop using screens, such as after sunset. You might also consider using blue light blocking glasses, a kind of nonprescription glasses that block blue light from technology from filtering to your eyes and brain. You can also change the settings on your phone and TV to emit warmer light.

Movement and Sleep Challenge

Beginner challenge: Go for a thirty-minute walk five times a week for one month. How do you feel afterward? Devote a night to the sleep test described earlier in this chapter. What does this tell you about changes you might want to make in your sleep schedule?

Intermediate challenge: Connect with a friend and commit to getting together to move your bodies once a week for the next month. Commit to leaving your phone outside your bedroom each night for a month. What differences do you notice about your sleep patterns and mental health?

Advanced challenge: Choose one movement style to try, and do it five days a week for a month. Determine what activity you'll do (get specific!), who you will do this activity with, what time of day you'll do it, and where it will take place. Be sure to have a backup plan if something like weather gets in your way. Create a nighttime routine that helps you calm your body and your mind before bed each night for a month. Write down the steps and check each one off as you complete them.

CHAPTER 4

THE PATH TO OPTIMAL FUNCTIONING

Keep your vitality. A life without health is like a river without water.

MAXIME LAGACÉ

On my own path to healing, I've learned that as vital as healthy eating is, that's not the only key to optimizing our health. In addition to being wise about what we're putting into our bodies, we also need to find—and heal—the root cause of illnesses. The healthy choices we make not only heal current conditions but also help our bodies function optimally to prevent future disease and dysfunction.

God's heart for us as his beloved children is to see us flourish. He doesn't just want us to survive; he longs for us to *thrive* so we can fulfill the purpose he has created us for. And while it's true that we live in a broken world where there is pain and illness, his desire is for us to live as healthy and whole as possible here on earth, until the day we experience complete healing in eternity. God's words recorded by Jeremiah reflect that desire: "I will give you back your health and heal your wounds" (Jeremiah 30:17, NLT).

The conventional method of disease management involves diagnosing a disease and then managing the symptoms. We are bombarded with pharmaceutical ads that tell us the next purple pill will solve all our problems. Instead of asking ourselves, *Why is this happening?* we tend to ask, *What could I take to make these symptoms stop?*

Functional medicine encourages a shift toward root cause analysis, which asks *why* in order to get to the underlying reason a disease or symptom is manifesting in your body. If you had a broken window in your home in the middle of winter, you would have the problem of a very cold home. There are things you could do to fix the undesirable circumstances you're experiencing. You could buy more comforters so you're warm while you sleep. You could max out your heating bill to try to keep your home warm. Or you could get to the root of the issue and replace the broken window, which would permanently solve your problem!

> We're not just working to minimize symptoms; we are looking for true healing and thriving.

If there's an aspect of our health that isn't functioning optimally, we need to explore why. It's also important to note here that there's a difference between common and normal. Just because a lot of people you know are experiencing a certain symptom (for example, maybe every mom you know is so exhausted they have to take a nap every afternoon or get a boost of caffeine just to make it through the day) doesn't mean that's normal and that you should be experiencing the same thing.

Our goal here is to optimize our health. We're not just working to minimize symptoms; we are looking for true healing and thriving. In chapter 2 we talked about putting good things in your body; in this chapter, we'll talk about how to support the detoxification process, or getting the bad things out. This is a major way to heal things that aren't working in your body now and prevent disease in the future. If you are experiencing any symptoms at all, I encourage you to work with a functional medicine practitioner to get to the root of the problem.

Healthy Hydration

Our bodies are made up of 55 to 75 percent water, so drinking water is clearly important. Staying hydrated is important for nearly every process in the body. It's needed to maintain electrolyte balance, aid digestion, disperse nutrients and oxygen throughout the body, regulate body temperature, deliver nutrients to cells, detoxify from unwanted substances, repair and energize muscles, cushion joints, and maintain function of the immune systems, which helps prevent infection.[1] Adequate hydration can also help you manage hunger, because sometimes what you think is a hunger cue is actually a sign that you need to drink more water. Proper hydration also improves the health and appearance of hair, skin, and nails. But as important as water is for the body, research indicates that almost half of Americans consume far below the recommended amount of water.[2]

Your liver and kidneys require adequate water to clean your blood, produce urine, and get rid of waste. Let's just say that if you're constantly dehydrated, things get sluggish! Water helps keep you regular, and regular stools are a major part of the detoxification process.

Interestingly enough, there is no one-size-fits-all formula for how much water you should drink each day. It depends on a number of factors, including your age, weight, activity level, and the other beverages you're drinking. Health organizations vary in their recommendations, from six to thirteen cups per day.

Because of over-farmed soil, we get fewer minerals in our food than previous generations did. Higher stress levels also lead our bodies to burn through minerals more quickly. As a result, almost all of us are low in nearly all minerals. Adding electrolytes into your water is a great way to get your daily dose of minerals. I like to add the LMNT brand electrolytes to my water throughout the day.

While the amount of water you drink is important, the type of water you drink might be even more important.[3] I used to think tap water had to be safe—after all, it's monitored and regulated by the government! Not so fast . . .

In recent years, many stories about city water have made headlines. In Flint, Michigan, so much lead was found in the tap water that a state of emergency was called.[4] The city of Chicago offered its citizens at-home testing kits to determine if there was lead in their drinking water. The results found that in a sample of almost three thousand homes, three out of ten homes "had lead concentrations above five parts per billion, the maximum allowed in bottled water by the US Food and Drug Administration."[5] In Chicago, many buildings have lead pipes that carry the water and leave residual lead in the drinking water—and in people's bodies. In Denver, where I live, I've seen billboards telling people to filter their water because of lead pipes.

Unfortunately, it's not just lead that's the problem, and it's not just Flint and Chicago.

The Environmental Protection Agency (EPA) currently regulates about ninety contaminants in drinking water. There are thousands of additional contaminants that aren't even measured, tested, or regulated. Some of these contaminants include pesticides, disinfection by-products, chemicals used in commerce, waterborne pathogens, pharmaceuticals, and biological toxins.

Each unregulated toxin has its own harmful consequences and side effects. One type of toxin in drinking water that isn't tested or regulated is called per- and polyfluororoalkyl substances (known as PFAS). They're also called "forever chemicals," because our bodies are incapable of breaking them down or detoxifying them, so they build up in the blood and organs. PFAS increase the risk of some cancers and can harm

Tips for Drinking More Water

- Try to drink water as your default beverage of choice.
- Start your day with a big glass of water or a cup of warm water with lemon or lemon essential oil to stimulate your liver.
- Set specific times throughout the day when you stop and intentionally drink water.
- Get a huge water bottle that helps you track your daily water intake. (I prefer toxin-free options like glass, silicone, or steel.)
- Always carry a water bottle with you and fill it up when you're on the go.
- Drink extra water when you're in hot, humid weather, when you're exercising, or when you're sick.

fetal development. The Environmental Working Group (EWG) suggests a reverse osmosis system (like the one we have from Aquasana) to get rid of PFAS in your water.

So how do you find out what's in your water?

How to Check Your Water Supply

Consumer Confidence Reports: First, you need to find out which water system provides your water. Most communal water systems participate in a Consumer Confidence Report (CCR) once a year. This report reveals where water is sourced and identifies contaminants and their possible health effects. You can search for yours at the EPA's website.[6]

Tap water database: Once you find out which water system provides your water, you can use the EWG's database to find results of water testing for that water system. Their database contains water records from 28 million samples collected in all fifty states. According to their results, about 80 percent of the water they tested contained chemicals that have been linked to cancer. They detected more than 250 contaminants, 180 of which the EPA hasn't set limits on. You can check their database using your zip code.[7] To give you an idea about the kind of information this source provides, the EWG found 34 contaminants for water in my zip code, 11 of which exceed the EWG health guidelines. The contaminants in my water include arsenic, chloroform, and radium—all of which have been identified as potential cancer-causing agents.

At-home water test: If the EWG database doesn't include your zip code in their database, if you're on well water, or if you want additional information, you can complete an at-home water test. You can use Varify's water test to check for seventeen contaminants, including bacteria, metals such as lead, nitrite, and nitrate. It also tests for alkalinity, hardness level, and pH level.

Choosing a Water Filter

I've never met anyone who searched the EWG Tap Water Database and found out that their water was completely clean, with no concerns. No matter where you live, it's likely that you need some kind of water-filtration system.

Best: Because toxins from water can get into the body through the skin while bathing, our family got a whole-house water system from Aquasana. It's a significant investment, but it's also something that provides long-term benefits, as it filters and cleans your drinking and bathing water for ten years.

Better: If a whole-house system isn't an option for you right now, another possibility is an under-sink system. I recommend the SmartFlow Reverse Osmosis under-sink system from Aquasana. It filters out 99 percent of ninety contaminants (this is fifteen times more than the leading gravity water pitcher). It filters out chemicals from the water treatment process such as chlorine, microplastics, asbestos, lead, mercury, chemicals, herbicides, pesticides, insecticides, fumigants, and pharmaceuticals.

Good: If you're on a tight budget, I recommend an Aquasana countertop water filtration system. They have options that can be installed in your showerhead as well.

The Truth about Bottled Water

So if tap water contains so many contaminants, is bottled water a better option?

We've been led to believe that bottled water is better than tap water. The reality, however, is that it's often just tap water put in a bottle.[8] Not only that, but consumers spend three hundred times the cost of tap water to drink bottled water. In just one year, the bottled water industry grossed $11.8 billion on 9.7 billion gallons of bottled water.[9] Bottled water is a booming business, but it's benefiting those who make it, not those who drink it.

Another downside of bottled water is the staggering environmental impact. Each plastic bottle takes up to one thousand years to degrade, and many of the particles left in the ocean are so minuscule that we won't know the true effects for generations.

So skip the bottled water and use filtered water in a glass or steel reusable water bottle instead!

Personal-Care Products

Similar to my assumptions about water, I assumed personal-care products were regulated by the government. I thought that if something was on a shelf in a store, that meant it had been evaluated, tested, and proven to be safe for my family and me. Unfortunately, regulations for these products are woefully outdated, though there has been a bit of progress in recent years.

You may wonder why it matters what you put on your skin or your hair. After all, it seems like the skin is a barrier. It is . . . to an extent. But chemicals pass the skin barrier and get into the body and even the bloodstream. A recent survey shows that on average, women use thirteen personal-care products a day, which translates to a total of more than a hundred different chemical ingredients that come into contact with our skin daily.[10]

On a daily basis, we face an onslaught of harmful toxins and chemicals. While it's true that our bodies are able to detoxify, they get bogged down by so many unhealthy substances. Think of it like a disposal in your kitchen sink. It's made to break down food particles and send them down the sink with ease. But let's say you started out with a few bites of cereal and milk and it went down easy-peasy! You thought, *Wow, this thing is magic! Let's see what it can do!* So you put in a four-pound beef brisket, a batch of mashed potatoes, and a whole bunch of asparagus. Would that work well? Probably not.

When we're talking about what our bodies can handle, it's really about capacity. The onslaught of chemicals overtaxes our bodies' detoxification system. And when this system gets overworked, it stops functioning optimally.

According to the EWG, US consumers are exposed daily to an average of two ingredients that are linked to cancer and two chemicals that can harm reproductive and development systems.[11] Two decades ago, the EWG created a massive database that evaluates the safety of personal-care products, and it now boasts more than 100,000 products. They analyze the safety of the ingredients and identify products that could be hazardous to your health.

But even with the help of resources like this one, it can be overwhelming to figure out what is safe and healthy for you and your family. The EWG alone has an "unacceptable" list that's hundreds of pages long.[12] To make matters more complicated, companies aren't even required to put the ingredients of their products on the label, so it can be hard to know what's even in the products you're buying.

If you're considering purchasing a product and you're not sure how it ranks in terms of safety, consider this: clean products will let you know. It is much more expensive to manufacture safe products than standard ones. So if a company has taken measures to create a nontoxic product, they're counting on that being its biggest selling factor. It won't be a secret. And if a product does not make these claims, there's a strong likelihood that it's not a clean product. This isn't a guaranteed method, and it's always a good idea to double-check safety. I know I've been tricked by greenwashing before—when companies make their products look like they're a healthy alternative when they're not really safe.

I recommend looking up products you purchase in the EWG Skin Deep database. Products are ranked one to ten for safety, with ten representing the highest level for concern. On the other end of the spectrum, there is the EWG VERIFIED category, which indicates products that meet their standards for health and transparency.[13]

> **Best:** If you have the budget to do an overhaul and replace your products with safer alternatives all at once, go for it!

Better: Most of my clients make the swap to safe products slowly, since this can be an expensive process. One way to do this is to replace items one by one as you run out of them. That makes more sense financially, and it's not as overwhelming to find all new products at one time.

Good: Choose one item at a time and switch to a healthier alternative. Start with the items that you use most frequently or that rank the worst in the Skin Deep database.

Supporting Your Body's Detoxification Systems

Our bodies have built-in systems to clear out waste and unwanted toxins. While our organs work together to do this automatically, there are things we can do to promote healthy functioning.

Promote Daily Bowel Movements

Your poop is actually a huge sign of your overall digestive health. If you're not pooping regularly, it can lead to a buildup of toxins in the body. According to Johns Hopkins Medicine, about 4 million people in the United States struggle with frequent constipation.[14]

If you're not experiencing daily bowel movements, there are things you can do to make that a reality:

- Exercise daily.
- Eat adequate fiber.
- Avoid low-fiber foods such as dairy until you get regular again.
- Hydrate with added electrolytes.
- Take digestive enzymes.
- Eat clean, whole foods.
- Prioritize eating foods high in magnesium and take it in supplement forms as well.
- Reduce stress, especially before and during mealtime.

Drink Organic, Cold-Pressed Juices

Drinking organic, cold-pressed juices has so many benefits. You're putting the nutrients of vegetables and fruits into a concentrated form. Of course, different fruits and vegetables produce varying amounts of juice. But to give you an idea, it takes about 1.6 pounds of produce to make just one sixteen-ounce serving of juice.[15]

Juice is a concentrated form of vitamins, minerals, antioxidants, phytonutrients, probiotics, and plant enzymes. Nutrients such as vitamin C and minerals can give you a boost of energy and improve your immune system. The cruciferous vegetables found in green drinks can also improve the liver's detoxification process, helping your body expel toxins more quickly.[16] I prefer to make my own juices using a juicing machine, or you can buy them from a local juice shop. There are also brands like Evolution Fresh and Suja that are available in grocery stores.

Some notes: Because of the high concentration of produce, it's important that your juices are organic to avoid harmful toxins. If you're struggling with metabolic syndrome, prioritize juices with more vegetables than fruits to reduce your sugar intake. Additionally, you can drink juice with or right after a meal instead of on its own, which would spike your blood sugar.

Drink Tea

Green tea and herbal teas are weak diuretics that promote kidney detox. Your kidneys' primary function is to flush toxins and other waste from your blood by turning it into urine once it has been cleaned by the liver.[17] Teas are able to stimulate this process gently. More importantly, tea contains polyphenols, antioxidants, and other components that may reduce the risk of cancer, cardiovascular disease, arthritis, and diabetes.[18]

Use Salt to Your Advantage

Breathing in salty air can improve breathing and keep your lungs free from infection and allergies, so let's head to the beach, shall we? If you aren't able to spend time by the ocean, you can visit a "salt cave" found in some spas or use a Himalayan salt inhaler at home to get the same effect.[19] Also called halotherapy, breathing in salty air infuses the respiratory system with beneficial minerals. This can be especially beneficial for those dealing with lung problems like asthma, bronchitis, and a cough of any kind.

Salt also helps with maintaining clear sinuses. You can use a saline mixture in a neti pot to treat allergies, colds, and congested sinuses.[20]

Take a Detoxification Bath

I absolutely love taking a detoxification bath—it's an easy and cheap at-home detox solution. While you can find many different recipes, most include a hot bath with Epsom salts, baking soda, and essential oils. Epsom salts aid in detoxification and have the added benefits of magnesium, a trace mineral that can be absorbed through the skin. Baking soda helps detox and alkalinize the body.

While the standard American diet tends to create an acidic environment in our bodies, an alkaline environment (more basic on the pH scale) is beneficial for many reasons: it can improve electrolyte ratios, benefit bone health, mitigate chronic diseases such as hypertension, increase growth hormone production (which can improve cardiovascular health and memory), and increase the presence of magnesium, which is required to activate vitamin D.[21]

Experts suggest that a detox bath should be up to one hour to give your body time to detox and take in the minerals from the Epsom salts. (This is a good solution if you love bath bombs but want to skip the icky chemicals!) You can choose your favorite essential oils or use oils with the therapeutic benefits you're looking for.

Dry Brushing

Dry brushing involves scrubbing with a stiff-bristled brush all over your body. A dry-brushing routine for the entire body requires as little as five minutes, so it's a quick, easy practice to add to your daily routine. The benefits of dry brushing include "stimulating the lymphatic system, exfoliating the skin, removing toxins, increasing circulation and energy, and reducing cellulite."[22]

To dry brush, start at your feet, and make short strokes toward your heart. Then brush your legs, followed by your abdomen (use a clockwise motion on the stomach). Then brush your arms. Because of the exfoliating nature of dry brushing, most people enjoy rinsing off with a shower afterward. Experts recommend dry brushing in the morning since it has some invigorating qualities.

Use a Sauna

Sweating is a method of detoxification. A traditional sauna gets hot and allows your body to detox simply through sweating. One study found sauna usage helps detoxify from heavy metals like arsenic, cadmium, lead, and mercury through the process of sweating.[23] An infrared sauna detoxifies on a cellular level. Infrared waves penetrate deep into the body's tissues, raising body temperature from the inside out. Proponents of infrared saunas claim it helps reduce pain, stimulate metabolism, increase detoxification, improve the cardiovascular system, destabilize cancer cells, and stimulate the immune system.[24]

There are near-infrared, mid-infrared, and far-infrared saunas, and each type emits a different type of infrared wavelength, with varied benefits. To receive the benefits of all three, seek out a full-spectrum infrared sauna. You can find infrared saunas you can pay to use, or you can invest in one for your home. We have the HigherDose infrared sauna blanket, and I love it! While it's still an investment, it's more affordable than a wooden, full-spectrum infrared sauna.

The Fiber Gap

The "fiber gap" refers to the fact that most people don't get enough fiber in their diet. In fact, 95 percent of Americans fall short of the Institute of Medicine's recommended daily fiber target.[25] According to these guidelines, women should get twenty-five grams of fiber per day and men should get thirty-eight grams.[26]

The consumption of fiber has dropped drastically in recent decades. This is due in part to the fact that high-fiber foods are being replaced with highly processed foods. On any given day, about 40 percent of Americans eat fast food, which is typically low in fiber.[27]

You've probably heard a lot of talk about fiber, but what exactly is it? According to the Mayo Clinic, dietary fiber includes the parts of plant foods your body can't digest. Unlike fats, proteins, or carbohydrates, which your body can break down and absorb, fiber passes through your stomach, small intestine, and colon relatively intact, and then is eliminated from your body.[28]

The Role of Fiber

Your body needs both soluble fiber (which dissolves in water) and insoluble fiber (which doesn't dissolve in water). Soluble fiber helps control blood glucose, which can reduce your risk for diabetes. Insoluble fiber helps promote bowel health and regularity.

There are many benefits to eating a diet rich in high-fiber foods (this includes the two main categories of fiber—both soluble and insoluble). Fiber helps you feel fuller for longer and helps reduce blood sugar spikes, which in turn helps you maintain a healthy weight. It also lowers your risk of diabetes, heart disease, and some forms of cancer. Dietary fiber can help feed the good bacteria in your gut,[29] and it can induce enhanced gut barrier function that protects the liver and kidneys.[30] It normalizes your bowel movements and helps you maintain bowel health. It lowers your cholesterol level and can even help you live longer.[31]

The reason we're talking about fiber in this chapter is because it aids in the detoxification process. Fiber binds either to toxins and heavy metals or to bile, which holds on to fat-soluble toxins to eliminate them from the body.[32] It's best to include a variety of soluble and insoluble fiber-rich foods into your diet for the greatest health benefits. When increasing fiber, also be sure to increase your water intake to prevent constipation.

One caveat about fiber: sometimes eating a high-fiber diet can make symptoms of irritable bowel syndrome worse (especially foods high in

Foods That Are High in Soluble Fiber

- Black beans
- Lima beans
- Brussels sprouts
- Avocados
- Sweet potatoes
- Broccoli
- Turnips
- Pears
- Kidney beans
- Figs
- Nectarines
- Apricots
- Carrots
- Apples
- Guavas
- Flaxseed
- Sunflower seeds
- Hazelnuts
- Oats
- Barley[33]

Foods That Are High in Insoluble Fiber

- Wheat bran
- Wheat germ
- Oat bran
- Beans
- Lentils
- Legumes
- Berries
- Whole grains (especially quinoa, sorghum, millet, amaranth, and oatmeal
- Turnips
- Green peas
- Okra
- Spinach
- Radishes
- Rutabagas
- Coconut
- Cocoa
- Apples (with skin)
- Pears (with skin)
- Flaxseed
- Avocados
- Sunflower seeds
- Potatoes
- Sweet potatoes
- Dried apricots
- Prunes
- Raisins
- Dates
- Figs
- Almonds
- Walnuts
- Passion fruit
- Pastas and breads (100 percent whole grain)
- Popcorn[34]

FODMAP carbohydrates, a group of difficult-to-absorb sugars). When increasing your fiber intake, start small and then add fiber incrementally to see how it goes. If you experience constipation or bloating, reduce your fiber intake for a while. If you struggle with IBS, try eating cooked fruits and vegetables as your fiber source.

Other Reasons for Detox

For the general population, the strategies in this chapter are sufficient for detoxification. That said, some people may have deeper health concerns that require detoxing with the help of a functional medicine practitioner. Examples include mold exposure, chronic infections like Epstein-Barr virus (EBV), candida overgrowth (which causes yeast infections), small intestinal bacterial overgrowth (SIBO), parasites, and heavy metals poisoning. In addition, some people may have underlying conditions such as insulin resistance, vitamin and mineral deficiencies, leaky gut syndrome, inflammation, or oxidative stress. A practitioner can identify any area of concern and provide a personalized plan for healing.

Detox Challenge

Beginner challenge: Hydrate! For thirty days, increase your water intake, adding electrolytes to make sure you don't flush the body of needed nutrients. (I love the LMNT brand.) Consider starting with 13 cups (or 104 ounces) for men and 9 cups (or 72 ounces) for women.

Intermediate challenge: Increase your fiber! For thirty days, follow the daily fiber recommendations from the Institute of Medicine. For women, aim for 25 grams of fiber per day. For men, shoot for 38 grams. I love this challenge, because it essentially means eating more vegetables and fruits! You will feel so much better as your increased produce pushes less nutritious foods off your plate.

Advanced challenge: Choose a detox practice and commit to it for thirty days. You might decide to drink organic, cold-pressed juices or herbal teas, or you might start taking detoxification baths. Maybe you can try halotherapy or the neti pot, or start dry brushing! Choose whichever practice you think would be most beneficial for you.

PART TWO

Environment

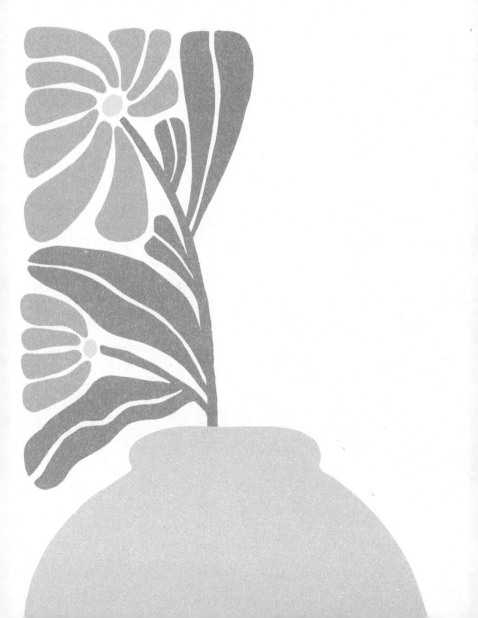

CHAPTER 5

HEALTHY HOME

The power of finding beauty in the humblest
things makes home happy and life lovely.
LOUISA MAY ALCOTT

My home is my sanctuary. It's where I make meals with my kids. It's where I've built more LEGO sets than I can count. It's where I've built bicycles on Christmas morning and kissed boo-boos later that afternoon. It's where we've hosted friends by the fire and cried tears on our pillowcases.

Our homes hold it all. And they should be our safe havens.

We are all born with an innate longing for home—both a home on earth and an eternal home. Proverbs 24:3 says, "A house is built by wisdom and becomes strong through good sense." A strong, healthy home isn't going to happen automatically; it's something we need to build with wisdom and intentionality.

We spend a considerable amount of time making our homes look beautiful, but are we also committed to making them havens of health?

When we think of pollution, we typically think of outdoor air pollution, mostly in major cities. But believe it or not, indoor air pollution is even more of a concern than outdoor air pollution. According to EPA studies, "Indoor levels of pollutants may be two to five times—and occasionally more than 100 times—higher than outdoor levels." This is especially concerning since most people spend about 90 percent of their time indoors.[1]

We spend a considerable amount of time making our homes look beautiful, but are we also committed to making them havens of health?

Many of the products we use contain unhealthy ingredients that can cause breathing problems, endocrine disruption, and even cancer.

We can be exposed to toxic substances in several different ways: by inhaling them (breathing them in via polluted air), through absorption (coming into contact with them through the skin and eyes), or ingestion (eating or drinking them).[2] In this chapter, we'll address the toxins in our homes that we're breathing in.

As we begin, you might want to head to Spotify and find that Anna Nalick song "Breathe (2 AM)" and use it as the soundtrack for the first part of this chapter. *Just breathe.* Unfortunately, that's easier said than done, because recent comparative risk studies performed by the EPA "have consistently ranked indoor air pollution among the top five environmental risks to public health."[3]

Why Does Indoor Air Quality Matter?

You might be thinking, *Okay, so the indoor air quality in most homes is pretty terrible. But why does that matter?* Great question! We breathe *a lot.* Did you know each person takes more than twenty thousand breaths in a single day? That number is even higher for babies and children.[4] Once chemicals get in your lungs, they end up in your bloodstream. Considering that your blood goes through your entire body, these chemicals can cause some widespread damage.

Having harmful indoor air quality (IAQ) can lead to both short-term and long-term health problems. Acute effects include coughing, sneezing, headaches, dizziness, nausea, fatigue, allergic reactions, short-ness of breath, and sinus congestion.[5] A poor IAQ can also trigger the onset or aggravation of asthma. The long-term effects of exposure to indoor pollutants are staggering and include respiratory diseases, endo-crine disruption, heart disease, and even cancer.[6]

Whether we realize it or not, anything we bring into our homes made with chemicals that leach into the air can negatively impact our indoor air quality. This includes household cleaners, candles, cooking pans, paints, mattresses, and furniture.

While detoxifying our home is about more than just air quality, breathing is one of the major ways we get chemicals into our bodies, so it's a good place to start. Fortunately, there's a lot we can do to make our indoor air fresh and clean!

Household Cleaning Products

When I was growing up, we had no idea that household cleaning prod-ucts could contain harmful chemicals. My family had a houseboat, and we used some serious cleaners to keep it spick and span. I specifically remember cleaning with Windex or 409 and thinking, *Man, this smells clean!*

We tend to think of heavy-duty cleaning products as being more effective because of their potency. But that chemical potency comes with some significant side effects. Let's talk about what's in traditional cleaning products. Well, it's actually hard to do that, because manufac-turers aren't required to list ingredients on their label as they are with food nutrition labels.[7] Not only that, but household products aren't required to be tested for safety for humans.[8] This is especially a concern for cleaning products, which often forego transparency under the guise of "proprietary trade secrets." Personally, I don't think any company's "secrets" should be harmful for humans.

According to the Environmental Working Group (EWG), only 7 percent of cleaning products adequately disclose their contents.[9] Most often, it's transparency that keeps companies honest and doing the right thing, so this lack of transparency results in products that contain terrible-for-you ingredients.

Household cleaning products can have a devastating effect on your indoor air quality—and your lungs. The EWG found that 53 percent of the cleaning products they evaluated contain ingredients known to harm the lungs, and 22 percent contain chemicals reported to cause asthma in healthy individuals. Suspected and known carcinogens such as formaldehyde, 1,4-dioxane, and chloroform are common ingredients in cleaning products. There are almost four thousand ingredients in household products that are categorized as "fragrance." These ingredients can cause allergies, skin irritations, breathing trouble, and reproductive harm.[10]

As with personal-care products, the labels of household products will indicate if they contain healthy, clean ingredients. I only purchase household products from companies that disclose their ingredients and list their toxic-free ingredients. You can check out the EWG's "Guide to Healthy Cleaning" to find healthy cleaning products. The EWG has an EWG verified label for household cleaners too. This label means the product is free from all the ingredients they've flagged for concern, the company has disclosed their ingredients, the product meets stringent air-quality standards, and the company uses good manufacturing practices.[11]

I like to use Branch Basics products in my home. They have a cleaning concentrate that is rated A by EWG, and they have oxygen boost and dishwasher tablets that are both EWG verified.

Volatile Organic Compounds

The Environmental Protection Agency describes volatile organic compounds (VOCs) as chemicals found in certain solids and liquids that emit gases. They are "compounds that have a high vapor pressure and low water solubility." VOCs contain various chemicals, including some that have "short- and long-term adverse health effects." VOC concentrations are higher indoors than outdoors (up to ten times higher!).

Thousands of different products emit VOCs, including paints, lacquers, paint strippers, cleaning supplies, pesticides, building materials, copiers, printers, glue, adhesives, and permanent markers.[12] Think of VOCs as that "new car smell."

If you need to paint, be sure to choose a nontoxic option. (My favorite brand is ECOS Paints.) There are low- and zero-VOC paints in most home-improvement stores. Look for products that are marked Greenguard Gold Certified, low VOC, or zero VOC. And whenever you can, paint outside instead of inside or open windows to get more airflow and circulation.

Plastic and BPA

Although you may not be able to smell it, plastics can emit gas just like VOCs. They also contain harmful ingredients, such as the hormone-disrupting chemical bisphenol A, or BPA. This chemical is harmful because it is a synthetic estrogen (meaning it mimics estrogen in the body). BPA has negative effects on our bodies, including "brain, behavioral, learning and memory impairment; cardiovascular abnormalities; diabetes; obesity; breast and prostate cancer; thyroid and sex hormone disruption; early puberty; changes to egg and sperm development and fertility; and genetic alterations that can be passed on to future generations."[13]

BPA is found mainly in hard plastics, thermal receipt paper, and epoxy resins, which is in the protective lining of food and beverage containers. (When you're getting food containers, look for the label "BPA free.") I refuse receipts or opt for digital ones when I can, because thermal paper has high concentrations of BPA.[14] According to the Environmental Working Group, retail workers have 30 percent more BPA in their bodies than the average adult.[15]

Avoiding plastics is top priority when it comes to items you're eating on, drinking with, or storing food in. (You can find a full list of tips for avoiding plastic in chapter 7.) I recommend materials such as glass, stainless steel, or silicone instead of plastic.

High-Toxicity Products to Avoid

- **Fabric softener and fabric sheets:** Fabric softener and fabric sheets often contain toxins that irritate the lungs and cause allergies or asthma. We use wool dryer balls instead, and I add a few drops of essential oils onto each ball for a nice scent. You can also attach a safety pin onto a wool dryer ball to release static.

- **Drain Cleaners:** According to Poison Control, consumption of drain cleaners can result in "serious burns, permanent tissue damage, and even death." [16] Sure, you're not going to intentionally take shots of drain cleaner, but even so, anything that can cause that kind of damage probably shouldn't be in your home at all. Instead of using traditional drain cleaner, you can manually remove a clog using a drain snake or use a "fizzy bath bomb" made from equal parts vinegar and baking soda. You can add lemon essential oil to combat grease buildup.

- **Oven Cleaners:** Like drain cleaners, oven cleaners can burn your eyes and skin.[17] Instead, use a mixture of baking soda, water, and lemon essential oil to scrub, degrease, and clean your oven.

- **Air Fresheners:** Fragrance is one of the most elusive ingredients, since these chemicals are often undisclosed and untested. They can trigger allergies and asthma, so I recommend skipping them and using an essential oil diffuser instead.[18]

- **Candles:** Candles are one of the biggest contributors to indoor air pollution. Most candles are made from paraffin wax, which contains petroleum and releases black soot when burned. This can exacerbate respiratory illness and disease. The fragrance in candles can also contain VOCs, formaldehyde, acetaldehyde, and other known carcinogens.[19] My favorite alternative to candles is an essential oil diffuser. You can make lovely fragrance combinations using your favorite oils. Not only are these not harmful, they also contain therapeutic benefits. If you're set on burning candles, make the switch to pure beeswax, soy, or palm oil candles, and be sure only natural fragrances are used.

Tried-and-True DIY Recipes

It's true that store-bought healthy cleaning products are typically more expensive than their conventional counterparts. But don't let cost hold you back from switching to cleaner products and creating a healthy home! I bought the ingredients for these recipes in bulk more than seven years ago, and I still haven't run out. Here are some of my favorite recipes to make at home.

All-Purpose Cleaner

Ingredients

1 cup white distilled vinegar
1 cup distilled water
½ teaspoon Sal Suds (available at most health food stores)
10 drops essential oils of your choice (I like doTerra On Guard, lemon, or wild orange)
16-ounce glass spray bottle

Instructions

1. Pour the ingredients into the 16-ounce glass spray bottle in the order listed. Gently shake the bottle to combine.
2. Spray on desired surface. Wipe the surface with a clean microfiber cloth.

Dish Soap

Ingredients

½ cup distilled water
1 tablespoon white distilled vinegar
½ cup Sal Suds
1 tablespoon olive oil (optional)
10 drops essential oils (I like lemon, wild orange, or grapefruit)
8-ounce glass bottle with a pump

Instructions

1. Using a funnel, pour the water and vinegar into the glass bottle.
2. Shake the bottle to combine.
3. Add the Sal Suds, olive oil, and essential oil, and gently shake the bottle again to combine. Bubbles may form—this is normal!
4. Use as you would typically use dish soap: a squirt for a sink of soapy water and a few drops per dish.
5. If the ingredients separate, shake before using.

Foaming Hand Soap

Ingredients

2 tablespoons liquid Castile soap (unscented)
1 tablespoon olive oil
10 drops essential oils of choice (I like doTerra On Guard or lemongrass)
Water
Glass bottle with foaming pump

Instructions

1. Pour the Castile soap and olive oil into the glass bottle.
2. Add the essential oils.
3. Slowly add water to the bottle, leaving room for the foaming pump.
4. Put lid on and shake.
5. Pump one to two squirts into hands and wash with warm water.

Stock Up with the Right Supplies

- **Microfiber towels:** These cloths trap bacteria in the rag, so you can use the cloth, rinse it, and use it over and over again. Not only are these better for the environment than paper towels, but they also are more effective at cleaning. We also have a microfiber pad on our mop that's washable and reusable, and it works great for cleaning our floors.

- **Abrasive brush:** When you need something to scrub away buildup, I recommend a steel wool cleaning pad. Just be sure it doesn't come with any cleaning agents inside. I find brushes like this helpful for hard-to-clean spots such as the oven or bathroom grout.

- **Squeegee:** For windows, mirrors, and glass, you'll get the best, cleanest shine using water and a squeegee.

- **Vacuum cleaner:** Since dust holds on to chemicals, I recommend a high-quality vacuum cleaner, especially if you have carpet in your home. A vacuum works better to catch and store dust than a broom, which returns dust from the floor into the air.

Quick Tips to Detoxify Your Home

It may sound overwhelming to detox your home, but it really can be simple! Here are some basic tips to make your cleaning products safe and effective.

- **Filter your water.** See chapter 4 for more on this topic.
- **Switch your dryer sheets for wool dryer balls.** If you prefer scented laundry, feel free to add essential oils.
- **Dust regularly.** Be sure to dust your home using a microfiber cloth. Aim to do this weekly.
- **Vacuum carpets regularly.** If you can, get a high-powered vacuum cleaner that comes with a high-efficiency particulate absorbing (HEPA) filter to absorb allergens and pollutants.
- **Swap out your regular candles.** You can use pure beeswax candles or essential oil diffusers instead.
- **Remove your shoes inside the home.** Since we're constantly walking on toxins (including E. coli), I recommend leaving shoes at the door.
- **Use a high-quality air purifier.** Be sure to vacuum air filters monthly and change the filters as indicated. We love our AirDoctor purifier.
- **Get high-quality HEPA-certified filters for your HVAC system.** Sometimes these are too thick to fit in your system, so get the highest quality that works for you.
- **Get your air ducts cleaned regularly.** Dust can settle in your air ducts and then move allergens and microorganisms such as pet dander, bacteria, pollen, mildew, and mold spores throughout your house. I recommend getting your air ducts professionally cleaned every two to three years.
- **Evaluate the materials you're cooking with, drinking from, and eating on.** I suggest using cast iron, enameled cast iron, stainless steel, or ceramic for your cookware and dishes. Try to avoid Teflon and plastics.

- **Avoid items with Prop 65 warnings.** These warnings refer to California's Proposition 65, which requires businesses to provide warnings about significant exposure to chemicals that may cause cancer, birth defects, or reproductive harm.
- **Avoid stain-resistant, UV-resistant, and flame-retardant chemicals.** These chemicals are often present on furniture, mattresses, and clothing. For furniture, look for solid wood, not MDF, which is made with wood particles and glue. Wood that's sealed with oil instead of sealant is ideal. Furniture companies don't have to disclose materials, but some do anyway. I look for companies that voluntarily disclose their materials. (We love our sectional from Medley.) Buying solid wood antique furniture is a great way to avoid buying new and increasing the demand for new goods, and it's a way to get high-quality pieces for your home at a lower price. You can also avoid furniture with a Prop 65 warning. For mattresses, get organic if you can. If you're looking for a foam mattress, consider CertiPUR-US, which is a certified foam made without toxic materials.
- **Swap the air fresheners in your home and cars.** Use an essential oil diffuser instead.
- **Don't buy anything that doesn't list the ingredients.** If the product doesn't overtly claim to be made with clean, safe ingredients, that's a sign you should probably find something else.
- **Look at the warnings.** I don't buy products that say "Keep out of the reach of children" or that include instructions for what to do if it's ingested or gets into the eyes. If it's harmful to the skin or body, then it's harmful to be in my home.
- **Evaluate before you buy.** Look for the EWG verified logo.
- **Make your own products.** Not only is this better for you and the environment, it's also cheaper!
- **Open your windows.** Most heating systems and air-conditioning systems don't bring in fresh air from outside. Instead, the same

air is circulated through your home over and over. On days when it's nice outside, open all your windows to get fresh air inside your home. Just be sure to check the outside air quality, and only open the windows if the air quality is good.

- **Use your fans.** Cooking is one of the biggest sources of indoor air pollution. Be sure that you turn on your downdraft fan when you're cooking on the stove. This removes the pollution from inside your home and takes it outside. In the bathroom, excess moisture can lead to mold, so be sure to turn on your bathroom fan anytime you take a shower or bath. If you have ceiling fans, run them on low to keep air flowing throughout your home.

- **Get houseplants.** A study by NASA found that indoor plants can remove VOCs from the air. Plants such as the lady palm, the parlor palm, and the peace lily remove benzene, formaldehyde, trichloroethylene, xylene, toluene, and ammonia.[20]

- **Make the switch to clean LED light bulbs.** See chapter 7 for more on this topic.

- **Block EMFs.** Electric and magnetic fields, also referred to as radiation, are associated with the use of electricity. EMFs come from microwaves, computers, Wi-Fi, cell phones, Bluetooth, power lines, and MRIs. Some people are more sensitive to EMF waves than others, but symptoms of EMF exposure include headaches, anxiety, depression, nausea, and insomnia.[21] You can get EMF-blocking devices for your phone, tablet, laptop, and headphones from companies like DefenderShield. You can also find products to protect your home from EMFs from places like SaticShield.

Clean Home Challenge

Beginner challenge: Make one of the DIY recipes for a cleaning product. Each time you use it, breathe easy with the knowledge that you're creating a safe sanctuary for your family.

Intermediate challenge: For the next thirty days, as you run out of cleaning supplies, make toxic-free replacements. Dust your home, vacuum, and open your windows once a week (if the weather allows!).

Advanced challenge: If your budget allows, do a clean sweep of your cleaning products and replace anything toxic all at once.

CHAPTER 6

SACRED SIMPLICITY

The things you own end up owning you.

FIGHT CLUB

When my family moved from Atlanta, Georgia, we found there's a very different culture in Denver, Colorado. In Atlanta, moms tended to be defined by their fashion and sense of style. The brands they chose were part of their identity. Many of them wore dresses from Nordstrom with Tory Burch sandals. Their children were dressed in smocked clothing. In Colorado, nearly everyone is defined by their dedication to adventure. It's Patagonia or bust. You'd better have a ski pass, own a kayak, and drive an electric car with four-wheel drive, or what are you even doing with your life?

No matter where you live or what the cultural norms are in your region, the same false assumption that what you have determines who you are drives people everywhere. This is the lie that repeats like a broken record: the more you get, the happier you'll be. We think we'll be happy when we get just a little more [fill in the blank with what you've been desiring: money, stuff, a home, a bigger home, a job, or a better job]. The list could go on.

But this is simply not true. When we get more, it only adds fuel to the fire. The more we get, the more we want. The satisfaction we're desiring never comes, and the desire for more only grows stronger.

It's a classic Eden situation on repeat. God provided Adam and Eve with everything they needed in the perfect Garden of Eden, but even so, they weren't satisfied and instead grabbed for that pomegranate (I like to think it was a pomegranate!). The same is true for us. We aren't grateful for what we have, and when someone suggests we should get that shiny new thing, we covet it like the forbidden fruit from the middle of the Garden.

Instead of taking God at his word, Adam and Eve replaced him with their desire to be God themselves. Likewise, we replace the Creator with his creation. We buy and consume in an attempt to satisfy us when no object or purchase ever will. This is idolatry at its most classic: worshiping things instead of the Creator of all things.

We are constantly bombarded with messaging that says we need more, more, more. On average, an American sees between 4,000 and 10,000 advertisements in a single day. This is especially staggering when you consider that in the 1970s, people were confronted with only 500 to 1,600 ads a day.[1] These ads are all aimed at our subconscious, subtly suggesting what we need to change to feel happier and what we should buy to feel fulfilled. When it comes to advertising, the United States spends the most money in the world by far, with a total of $250 billion going toward ads in a single year.[2]

So what's the result of all this advertising? We pull out our credit cards, and we buy. In fact, we buy so much that instead of purging what we already have, we purchase bigger homes. In 1949, the average size of a single-family home was 909 square feet. The average home in the US is now 2,480 square feet.[3] And even so, our stuff doesn't fit in our homes! The US now boasts more than 50,000 storage facilities—that translates to 5.9 square feet of storage space per American![4]

What Is Minimalism?

Minimalism can go by many names: simplicity, simple living, or frugality (this is what monks call it). Minimalism is consciously choosing less so we can experience more.

While minimalism does refer to the stuff in our homes, it's more than that. It's about our spending habits, the purchases we make, the way we spend our time, and the people we spend our time with. It is not just about how many knickknacks we have on our shelves; it's an entire mindset.

Minimalism may be a trend in the wider culture right now, but it actually has spiritual roots. Simple living is a spiritual discipline that was encouraged by Jesus himself. In his teaching, Jesus often taught with parables, and almost half of them dealt with the topic of money. In fact, nearly 15 percent of everything Jesus said had to do with money and possessions! The only topic he brought up more was the Kingdom of God. Jesus talked about money so much because we can easily turn to wealth to give us that sense of security only God can provide.

> Minimalism is consciously choosing less so we can experience more.

Matthew 6:24 says, "No one can serve two masters. Either you will hate the one and love the other, or you will be devoted to the one and despise the other. You cannot serve both God and money." We can't try to keep up with the Joneses while also being fully devoted to God.

It may feel like a stretch to think of simplifying your life as a spiritual discipline. But as we prioritize our lives and buy less, we seek to match our desires to God's desires. Romans 12:2 says, "Do not conform to the pattern of this world, but be transformed by the renewing of your mind. Then you will be able to test and approve what God's will is—his good, pleasing and perfect will." The pattern of this world is to buy more and have more to be more. In contrast, having less through the practice of sacred simplicity helps us focus on what is most important in our lives.

It helps me remember that regardless of what I have or don't have, my family and my relationship with God are the most important parts of my life.

Spiritual disciplines act as counterweights to the negative and pervasive effects of the culture around us. In a world that encourages consumerism, simplicity helps us counteract our consumeristic tendencies. In a world that tells us there's an endless list of things we need, simplicity helps us determine what a true need is.

Simplicity offers us freedom from the endless cycle of wanting more. It's not just about subtracting; it's also about adding. As we release our grip on stuff, we say yes to contentment, gratitude, peace, and joy.

What Will You Say Yes To?

If we want a lifestyle of minimalism to stick, we need to figure out what we're simplifying *to*. What is important to us and the culture of our family? In order to say no, we also have to figure out what we're saying yes to.

One way to determine your values is to do some self-evaluation. The way we spend our money is a huge sign of where our priorities are. As Jesus said, "Where your treasure is, there your heart will be also" (Matthew 6:21).

In order to say no, we also have to figure out what we're saying yes to.

Our family has two core values of faith and health—these are the priorities that form the foundation for every decision we make. We also deeply value generosity and family time. When we look at our budget, we try to align it with these values. For us, that means eating healthy, organic foods, taking supplements, taking care of our bodies, and using clean products. Chaz and I wake up early to have our quiet times, we prioritize going to church and serving on different teams on Sundays, and we are active on the leadership team of our church. We donate to our church, missionaries, and organizations we're passionate about. We spend money creating family memories like traveling and going skiing.

Each person—and each family—has different values. That's why it's important to be intentional about what is most important to you. You want to ensure that you're making choices based on what you value, not what someone else thinks you should do or what's important to them. If you're not sure what values are most central for you, I recommend choosing just two words that reflect your family culture most accurately and will guide future decisions. Of course, there will be many values that you believe in, but it simply isn't possible to focus on all of them at once.[5]

We've found that knowing our family values is our true north. Decision making is so much easier when we sift choices through our values first. Let me give you an example.

During my son's soccer season, there was a fire in another state that was making our air quality in Colorado terrible. The weekend of Owen's soccer tournament, the report was basically, "The air quality today will negatively affect anyone who is outdoors for any length of time. The elderly and children in particular should not go outdoors, and no effort-inducing activities such as sports should be done outside."

To our surprise, the games weren't canceled. I did some research and found that breathing air like this was essentially the same as smoking three to four cigarettes. I knew we couldn't let Owen play soccer outside in these conditions. It was hard because I knew how much he wanted to play in the tournament, but I sat Owen down and explained the situation. I told him it was a bummer because the soccer organization should have made a healthy choice for everyone involved. Instead, we had to opt out. While he was upset (at the situation, not at me), I made sure he understood our family value of health and why choosing not to play was in line with this value.

Saying no to having more and buying more allows you to prioritize what you value. It means you'll have more time, money, and mental capacity for the things that are most important to you.

My (Unexpected) Journey to Minimalism

I am not, by nature, a minimalist. After all, I'm an Enneagram 7, which means I love *more*—more things, more travel, more food, more pleasure, more fun! The idea of less isn't woven into my DNA.

If you're tempted to skip this chapter after seeing the word *minimalism*, I implore you to stick with me. No one is going to force you to get rid of everything you own (or even a single thing, if you don't want to!). As with the rest of this book, this chapter is intended to help you to become intentional in a way that resonates with you and the rhythms of your family.

Minimalism was "highly suggested" to me by my then-boyfriend (now-husband) Chaz when we were dating. While there are some minimalism evangelists who enjoy showing off their fashionable ten-piece capsule wardrobe and blogging about minimalism, this is not a trend for Chaz. It's a lifestyle. For as long as I've known him, he's been all about spending the least amount of money possible, and he craves simplicity.

In college, he was eating nearly exclusively black beans and pasta. He had lots of options there: black beans on their own, pasta on its own, or sometimes he would even *mix them*. He had a capsule wardrobe before that was even a term. He owned (and still owns) one or two items of clothing in every category. Jeans? One pair. Slacks? One pair. Tennis shoes? One pair. T-shirts? He splurges and has *two*. (Can you believe the audacity?)

On the other hand, I remember packing for my freshman year of college with my friend Addie. She looked through my closet in disbelief. How could I have so many clothes? At one point she asked if I wanted to get rid of some things because they didn't fit anymore. I'd argue, "But I wore that to the Coldplay concert!" or "But that was my first-kiss tank top!" At that point in my life, the memories and emotions surrounding my clothes were all-important.

I started dating Chaz at the beginning of my sophomore year, and that's when his minimalistic lifestyle choices started influencing my own. Instead of always going out to eat, he suggested we cook meals together.

He purposefully told me I was beautiful when I was in lounge clothes and no makeup. (He says he legitimately prefers the no-makeup look—I still don't get it!)

After a while, I started appreciating the simplicity of minimalism and began adopting the practices myself. Plus, after two years of sharing one hundred square feet with a roommate, I was starting to see the benefit of owning less stuff. To this day, I find that the amount of clutter around me is a direct reflection of the clutter in my brain. If my room or home is super messy, I'm also probably in a pretty high-stress season. It's kind of a chicken-or-egg scenario. While a stressful season tends to result in a cluttered home, I have found that the opposite is true too. If I'm feeling stressed and my home is cluttered, taking the time to purge, reorganize, and tidy up helps me feel calmer inside.

Now that we are married and have a family, I see the benefit of minimalism more than ever. Kids bring with them *stuff*—all the time and from everyone and everywhere. Practicing minimalism as a family is both a way to keep that constant clutter under control and a spiritual discipline that can help our children now and when they have their own homes one day!

We often think of minimalism as only being about our stuff, but it goes way beyond that. It's also a way to unclutter our hearts and minds so we have room for what we truly value.

How to Simplify Your Life

Once you've seen the ugly beast of consumerism for what it is and you're ready to live a life of sacred simplicity, the next question is *how*. Regardless of where you are on this journey, I recommend that you start slowly. This is a marathon, not a sprint!

In my experience, it's easiest to start with spaces in your home with the least emotional connection. I also recommend starting with a small space. You'll get done in a short amount of time, and it will give you the momentum to keep going and move on to other areas.

Remember that this is a new lifestyle, and it won't be a one-and-done situation. Our family goes through this process two or three times a year, because even with paring down our purchasing, things just tend to accumulate. The following process can be done in any area of your home and can be used over and over to maintain simplicity in your spaces.

Step 1: Keep or Purge

You can use the same process to simplify every room, area, or piece of furniture. First, you take everything out of every nook and cranny of that area. This is so you can see everything at once, and once it's out, you deal with it. The hardest part of the process is deciding if you want to keep or purge something. Purging can mean selling it, donating it, gifting it, recycling it, or throwing it away. I recommend getting eight boxes or piles per space: keep, wait, patch, sell, donate, gift, recycle, or trash.

Sometimes you just can't decide whether to keep something or not. You wonder if you'll regret getting rid of it, or you think you might need it sometime in the future. Put these items in the wait box, and set the box aside for a predetermined period of time—maybe six months, although the amount of time is totally up to you. During that period, if you need something out of the box, there's no shame! Just retrieve the item from the box. You might be surprised to discover at the end of the allotted time that you didn't need any of the items you tucked away. Now you can get rid of anything you didn't need and keep the things you used.

It's amazing how much money you can make on Craigslist or Facebook Marketplace selling your things. If we're running low on "fun money," I'll purge some belongings we don't need anymore so we can do something as a family with the money from the sale. I also sell clothes the kids have outgrown and use that money toward their new wardrobe.

Step 2: Patch

As a society, we have lost the skill of mending. When something is broken, we typically throw it away and replace it instead of fixing it. I have made it a goal for myself to repair more things. For me, this started by keeping a repair bin in our linen closet. I got a cheap sewing kit that includes everything I need: different sized needles, a thimble (I just love this word!), measuring tape, fabric scissors, and lots of different colors of thread. Now when an item of clothing gets a hole in it or when a seam rips, I fix it myself. I was even dubbed "mom of the year" when I managed to sew up a stuffed animal that was spewing out stuffing!

There may be things you don't know how to fix but someone else probably does. For as long as Chaz and I have been together, we've made it a habit to get our shoes resoled instead of getting new ones. The shoes feel as good as new, and for nicer leather shoes, the cost is about one-fourth of a new pair. Repairing things saves me money, and it means fewer things end up in a landfill—it's a win-win!

Step 3: Put It in Its Place

Once you decide to keep something, you will want to find a permanent home for it. If something is usually strewn about or not in its proper place, that's probably a sign it needs a permanent home—or a better one.

We live in Colorado, and it can get *cold* here. In the winter, the kids usually take beanies and gloves to school. I found that said beanies and gloves would be strewn about anywhere and everywhere when they got home—on the floor in the back entryway, on the back bench, or on the floor of the coat closet. I kept getting frustrated, but then I realized that we didn't have a true home for our winter gear. So I invested in a cubicle organizer. Each member of the family has their own cubby, and in the winter it holds their beanies, gloves, and scarves. In the summer it holds their hats, sunglasses, and goggles. Sometimes you just need to find the right system to keep things out of sight and out of mind.

Purging Tips, Room by Room

Bathrooms

Once you take everything out, look at your medications, makeup, and skin-care products. Check for expired products and toss them. One pro tip is to get a Sharpie and mark on the bottom of your makeup and skin-care containers the date you open them. Most people don't know this, but many cosmetics have a little icon that tells you the expiration date for the product. For example, "6M" would mean it expires six months after opening. That's helpful, but only if you know the date you opened it!

The most important question to ask yourself about these products is "Do I actually use this?" If you haven't used something in six months or more, you don't need to hang on to it thinking you might use it in the future. (The only caveat here is if you order multiples of things when they're on sale. In this case, you can have a back-stock section of your bathroom where you keep your extras.)

This is a great time to purge personal-care products that contain toxins. A note as you're purging: if something isn't safe for you, it's also not safe for someone else. For that reason, I toss toxic products instead of donating or gifting them. If bottles are recyclable, they will have a recycle symbol on them.

Once you've decided what you want to keep, put the things you use daily in an easy-to-access drawer or shelf. I have a little tray with all my daily items in it so I can pull them out, use them, and then put them away.

Bedroom

To simplify your bedroom, I recommend starting with your bedside table. (The closet is typically a massive project, so we'll tackle it separately.) The bedside table can accumulate a lot of items that don't need to be there. Once you've removed everything, put away anything that doesn't live there, like those seven glasses that really belong in the kitchen (speaking from personal experience here). Remove any books that you've finished or that you've had in your to-read pile but—let's be honest— you're not going to read. Put them back on your bookshelf for another time. You want your bedside table to be clear on the top, and the drawer should just contain things you genuinely need around bedtime. That may include your reading glasses, blue-light blocking glasses, an eye mask, earplugs, and any supplements you take at night. Don't let this be a place where things come to die!

Put anything that deserves to be on your bedside table in its rightful place. You'll be amazed how much better you feel when you go to sleep and wake up in an uncluttered space. The act of decluttering itself gives you endorphins (yes, the happy neurotransmitters you get after exercising!), and a clutter-free space is less distracting and improves focus.[6] For me, a clean bedroom helps me feel calm, which is a great vibe for a place that is mostly used for sleeping!

Office/Papers

Going through the papers in your home can feel totally overwhelming, because papers can pile up anywhere and everywhere. Paper clutter might be one of the worst types of clutter because it often includes action items, such as bills to pay, papers to organize, and permission forms to sign. But trust me, when you get done, it's so rewarding!

An obvious perk is that your surfaces are free of all the things! And you no longer have the mental drain of seeing those bills and deciding over and over if this is the time to tackle them. The first step in decluttering and organizing your papers is to get them all out. I'm talking all of them, from everywhere. Look around your home and note where the papers tend to stack up. This may be an indication that you need a system for that kind of paperwork. (More on that below.)

Now it's time to tackle your paperwork! The piles are a bit different when it comes to papers:

- **Keep:** Choose an organization system for the paperwork you need to keep. We have a file folder box for this purpose. We designate one file for each member of the family. This includes documents such as medical records, birth certificates, and passports. Then we have one file for our home, one for our cars, and one for each year of our taxes (more on that below).
- **Action:** When I'm going through paperwork, I often find there are things I need to do, whether that's a bill that needs to be paid or a receipt for something that needs to be returned. Put anything associated with an action you need to take in this pile.
- **Trash:** Sometimes I find things in my "paper" piles that aren't actually paper and need to be thrown out. So keep a trash can nearby in case that proves true for you too.

- **Recycle:** If it doesn't contain sensitive information and you don't need to keep it, recycle it!
- **Shred:** This pile is for anything with personal information on it.
- **Taxes:** This pile is for anything you need for your taxes. It's important to keep tax records in case you get audited, even years down the road. The IRS suggests keeping pertinent records for three years from the date you filed your original return or two years from the date you paid the tax (whichever is later). Keep records for seven years if you filed a claim for a bad debt loss.[7] (But keep in mind, I am no accountant! Be sure to check with a certified public accountant to determine what you personally need to keep, especially if you have complicated taxes.)

It's possible to go digital with almost all of your paperwork to declutter your space. Simply download a scanning app on your phone and take pictures of your files. After they're scanned, you can recycle or shred the papers! There are plenty of apps that keep these files in the cloud in case something happens to your phone.

The exceptions are when you have a document with a lot of pages, such as loans and tax information. Personally, I'd rather stash all those home-loan papers than scan them.

After you've sorted your paperwork, how do you ensure this paper clutter doesn't happen again? As I mentioned earlier, the key is to create a process for incoming paperwork. I suggest having a sort of "mailbox" in your home where you put any papers that you need to sort. When you get your mail, go ahead and recycle any junk right away. Then you're left with action items or mail for specific people. One way to keep track of your papers is to have a standing paper organizer for each member of your family (or just the adults, if your kids don't get mail often). You could also have one for incoming mail and one for outgoing mail. You can also add one for "action," meaning it's something you need to take care of, such as a bill.

Paperwork: Keep or Toss?

- **Receipts:** If the return period is over and you're keeping the item you bought, toss the receipt. If you need to return the item, put the receipt in the "action" pile. (And remember, as we discussed in chapter 5, try to refuse receipts as much as possible. Opt for electronic or skip it altogether to avoid hazardous BPA. Fewer receipts will make this process even easier the next time you do it!)

- **Bills:** When I pay a paper bill, I almost always write "paid" with the date on the bill, scan it in an app (I use Genius Scan), and toss it. You don't have to scan it if you have a digital copy in your online account.

- **Letters:** I personally don't keep cards, especially birthday cards that are only signed. I keep longer letters if they have sentimental value. How much to get rid of here is up to you!

- **Instruction manuals:** For newer appliances, manuals are now available online 99.9 percent of the time. Do a quick search to see if you can find the manual in question online, and if so, recycle the paper copy. If not, find a place for these instruction manuals to live all together.

- **Coupons:** First, ask yourself, Do I actually use coupons? Seriously, do you go to the grocery store, buy the thing you have a coupon for, and then hand the coupon to the checkout person? If the answer is no, go ahead and recycle those coupons and give yourself permission to never clip another one in your life. If you do use coupons, toss the expired ones. Then use a system such as an accordion organizer to store them so they're not all over the place and so you can easily find them when you need them.

- **Medical records:** I scan our medical records in an app designed specifically for this purpose. I also recommend scanning documents that relate to insurance, an FSA, or an HSA.

- **Magazines:** Did you read it? Great—you can recycle it now! Haven't read it? Is it from this month? Nope? Are you actually going to read it? If not, it's fine to get rid of it.

Kitchen and Pantry

The kitchen may feel daunting since there's so much to sort through, so you may want to break it into several stages—for example, appliances, dinnerware, serving dishes, drinkware, utensils, cutlery, and cleaning supplies.

The kitchen is the room I spend the most time in (besides my bedroom, of course!). Cooking is my thing, and I love my gadgets and appliances. But even so, it pays to simplify your kitchen, because minimizing your appliances, tools, and gadgets helps you streamline your cooking process. You might not need that miniature waffle maker that takes about four hours to make enough waffles to feed your family . . .

Simplifying your appliances to just an air fryer, a high-powered blender, and an Instant Pot might cut down on decision fatigue. You might find some fabulous recipes that work well for those appliances and free you up from worrying about the rest.

How to Handle Kids' Schoolwork and Artwork

A note on kids' schoolwork and artwork: there are barrels and buckets of this stuff! In my experience, the sheer bulk of art creation starts to decrease after kindergarten. When Owen was done with kindergarten, I took all my kids' artwork, photographed it, and made a little book out of it using Chatbooks. It takes up about one percent of the space that all their artwork took up, and I appreciate it just as much. An added bonus was that I had books made for all the grandparents for Christmas that year, and they were a hit! Here's your permission slip to document and toss your kids' art. When it comes to kids' schoolwork, I keep things like progress reports, but only if that data isn't otherwise available to me on a website. Papers like math homework get the toss when we're done with them.

Go through your kitchen, drawer by drawer, cabinet by cabinet, and ask yourself if you've used this appliance, gadget, or dish in the past six months. If the answer is no, donate it right away or put it in a wait box for six months to see if you end up using it. Put a date on the box, and if you haven't used it in that time, donate the whole box (try to resist the temptation to peek in the box!).

The next step is to simplify your pantry. Throw out anything that is expired or donate anything you realistically aren't going to use. You can also use this time to "healthify" your pantry, getting rid of foods in the "sometimes" or "never" category that you don't want to eat anymore. I recommend taking everything out of the pantry and evaluating whether you want to keep it. If you decide to keep it, put it back in the place that makes the most sense. As with your bathroom cabinets, you can reserve one area of your pantry for immediate use and another less accessible area for extras.

Living Room

Depending on where your living room or family room is, it can become a dumping ground for everyone's stuff! As I'm simplifying this room, my mantra is "Only things that belong in the living room stay in the living room." When you find things that belong to the other people, make a pile for each family member. When you're done, it can be their job to put away their things, if they're old enough to do so. Even young children can learn to take ownership of their things, so try to involve them in this process early!

If you have lots of different pieces of furniture, such as a bookshelf, a coffee table, and a media center, you might want to tackle one at a time. Remove anything you don't use anymore (DVDs can be a big one here!). If you own DVDs for movies that are available on your streaming platform, go ahead and donate them. Anything you use in this room can stay; anything that isn't used in the living room must go!

A note on books: if you love to read (like I do!), it might be time to pare down your books. I personally like to keep books that were formational for me so other people can borrow them—almost like my own intentional-living, health-and-wellness library. If your bookshelf is overflowing with books, try to remove any you won't read or reference again or won't be loaning to others.

Entryway/Mudroom/Foyer

Whether or not you have an actual foyer, you definitely have a place where you enter your home. And from my experience, this space can get cluttered *fast*. Keeping this area organized is mission critical. Why? Because we lose a lot of stuff—most of which lives in the entryway! According to a lost-and-found survey, Americans spend 2.5 *days* a year looking for lost items and $2.7 billion annually replacing things we've lost![8]

Rule number one for my family when it comes to the entryway: no shoes in the house. Shoes carry in the dirt from outside. Along with dirt, shoes also carry E. coli, a nasty bacteria you don't want in your home.

Since we ask people to remove their shoes when they come in, we have a shoe rack in our entryway coat closet. In the wintertime, since it snows in Colorado, we also have a large rubber mat to put shoes on. This kind of organization can be helpful not just for your guests' shoes but also for your own family's shoes. We have a cubby where each family member stores their shoes, and it makes getting out the door much easier!

Another trick is to keep your socks near the door instead of with your clothes. It's an extra step when putting away your laundry, but it saves time when you're leaving the house.

Have a specific place where your keys live, ideally right by the door you use to enter your home. We have hooks installed right next to the door.

I learned from Marie Kondo's book *The Life-Changing Magic of Tidying Up* to empty my purse every time I come home.[9] While this might be quite an undertaking the first time you do it, it shouldn't take much time after you start doing it daily. Keep your purse by the door for easy access.

Kids' Rooms

Since kids are constantly growing and changing, it's helpful to simplify their rooms regularly. I like to do this each season, or at least twice a year, which corresponds to when I look through their clothes. We do a "fashion show," where I get them to try on clothing for the upcoming season. We donate anything that doesn't fit (we try to think of friends we could give hand-me-downs to), and they can let me know if there are items they don't like anymore. Then I take inventory of what we have and what we need to fill out their wardrobes.

We also take this time to go through other things in their rooms—mainly toys. The biggest question we ask our kiddos is "Do you actually play with this?" If the answer is an emphatic "Yes!" but you know that it's actually a clear no, we use the wait box with them too. I tell my kids, "Okay, we can keep this toy for now. But I want you to remember this moment, and when we purge your toys again, if you still haven't played with it, we'll give it away."

While there are lots of different strategies to help kids purge their belongings, I think the most important part is to make sure they're involved. They won't learn simplicity if you sneak into their rooms and get rid of a bunch of their toys without their noticing. You might be minimizing their things, but they won't be learning the skills of purging or being generous.

When Ella Rae was five years old, we purged a bunch of her books. We went through her bookshelf together and decided to give some books to friends and some to a secondhand store. Less than a month later, I walked into Ella Rae's room, and she was staring at her bookshelf. I asked her what she was doing, and she said, "Mommy, I still have too many books. There are some I don't really read anymore, and there are lots of kids who can't afford books. I would like to give some of my books to them." Cue. The. Tears. When we practice these habits with our children, they learn to embrace simplicity themselves.

Garage/Yard

Go through your garage just like you would other areas in your home, and pull everything out. Once you're done sorting into the typical piles, you can decide if you need an organizational system to keep your garage tidy. We have pantry-style shelves and put large Rubbermaid containers on them for things like painting and gardening. We also have small plastic containers with drawers for items like nuts, bolts, and screws.

This is a good time to talk about the concept of community sharing. In our neighborhood, we all have postage-stamp yards. We live in a townhome, and some of our neighbors have about forty-eight square feet of lawn to mow. It seems silly for all of us to have lawn mowers when there is such a small amount of grass to cut. Have you ever thought about how much sense it would make if we could share the things we own? Find neighbors who have supplies that will complement yours, and you can share your supplies and appliances with each other. You can also rent single-use tools at home-improvement stores. If you'll only need that paint sprayer for one day, it might make more sense to rent it instead of buying it and storing it.

Closet

Most of us have a closet brimming with clothes, many of which we rarely wear. That's why I recommend a capsule wardrobe—meaning you have few items of clothing and most of them go together. The key is to find pieces that you love, look great on you, and make you feel like a million bucks (at least, that's the goal!).

Opinions vary on how many items should be in a capsule wardrobe, but I say the fewer the better. The idea is to get your wardrobe down to what you need and minimize excess. I like to think about my wardrobe in terms of the purpose it's fulfilling. There are lots of things I have one of: a raincoat, a winter coat, tennis shoes, sandals, and waterproof boots that work in rain or snow. Even if you love fashion, I would still encourage you to minimize your wardrobe. Consider making a capsule wardrobe of the essentials and then add in more fun/stylish pieces.

The idea of minimizing your wardrobe may feel limiting at first. You might wonder, *What will people think of me if I show up in the same outfit?* News flash: people really don't care what you're wearing! Realizing this was freeing for me.

Luke 12:27-28 says, "Consider how the wild flowers grow. They do not labor or spin. Yet I tell you, not even Solomon in all his splendor was dressed like one of these. If that is how God clothes the grass of the field, which is here today, and tomorrow is thrown into the fire, how much more will he clothe you—you of little faith!" This passage highlights why minimizing our closets can have a holy connotation. The fewer things we have to worry about and think about, the more capacity we have to think about God and his Kingdom.

I have some specific guidelines for purging your closet. You want your clothes to make you look and feel beautiful, right? So after you pull everything out of your closet (and anywhere else you have clothes), try things on. If you struggle with self-esteem and confidence (or if you feel like you don't really know whether something looks good on you), you might need a friend for this phase. Pick someone who is both decisive and kind. You want someone who will say, "Ehhh, I think those other jeans fit better"—telling you the truth without adding to your body image issues! If you have clothes that no longer match your life phase, get rid of them. Also get rid of anything that still has tags but hasn't been worn. Don't let guilt get hold of you. If you haven't worn it since you bought it, you're not going to. (And just think of the person who will be so excited to find a brand-new item at a secondhand store!)

I find it's easiest to take one category at a time. Compare all items and just keep your favorites in each cate-gory. I donate anything that I don't want anymore but is still in good condition. Anything with stains or holes I put in a clothing recycling pile. It might sound strange to recycle clothing, but there are places that do just that! You can do an online search to find clothing recy-cling drop-offs near you. If there are items you want to sell, you can use ThredUp, Poshmark, or Facebook Marketplace. I especially love selling clothes and then using that money to buy other clothing or accessories I need.

One caveat here: if you want to keep clothes you love but don't fit you anymore (whether they're too big or too small), you can keep them in a separate storage area. When these clothes that don't fit are in view, it adds to decision fatigue. Let's make it easier on ourselves, shall we?

> ## Questions to Consider When Purging Your Closet
>
> - Do you love it?
> - If you saw this on a rack at a store, would you buy it now?
> - Does it look great on you?
> - Does it fit well (now, not at the size you hope to be in the future!)?
> - Is it comfortable?
> - Is it still in good condition (no stains, no holes, etc.)?
> - Is this your favorite item in this category?
> - Does this work with other things you already have?
> - Have you worn this during the season it was appropriate in (or within the last six months)?

Once you've decided what you want to keep, put those pieces back in your drawers and closet. If you want to track which clothes you're wearing, you can get a spool of ribbon and cut it into six-inch strips. Each time you wear something, put a ribbon on the hanger and move it to the right side of your closet. After three to six months, you'll be able to identify anything you're not actually wearing.

Questions to Ask Yourself before Buying Something

- Do you actually *need* this?
- If this is a want and not a need, could you wait two weeks to make sure you really want it?
- Is there something you already have that could fulfill this same need or purpose?
- Have you gotten something similar before that you ended up not using or loving?
- Is this purchase in line with your values—with who you are and what you care about?
- Do you want to put in the time, effort, and budget to maintain this thing?

Questions to Ask Yourself Once You've Decided to Buy Something

- Could you buy it used somewhere to make it more affordable and better for the planet?
- Is it worth buying the highest quality of this thing so you don't have to replace it soon?
- Can you find a handmade or fair-trade version of this item?
- Is the thing you're buying beneficial (or not harmful) for your health and the planet's health?
- What will happen when you're done with this thing? Can it be reused in another way? Can it be recycled, or will it go in a landfill?

Phone Simplicity

Have you ever stopped to think how strange it is that we walk around with tiny computers in our pockets? Many applications for our phones, especially social media, were made to be addictive, so it's easy to spend way too much time on our phones. We often see more information within the first few hours of waking up than our grandparents saw in a week! This much cell phone usage can lead to mental clutter and anxiety. Try to simplify your cell phone usage with these tips:

- Keep your cell phone out of your bedroom.
- Spend a chunk of time in the morning without your phone.
- Remove as many notifications as possible.
- Delete any apps you don't need or use.
- Set goals for your screen time usage and monitor it weekly.
- Set screen time limits for your apps.

- Cut down on your news intake and catch up just once weekly.
- Follow fewer people on social media.
- Put your phone in a drawer when you get home.
- Put your phone away during meals and family time.
- Designate certain activities for your computer only (like checking email or social media).
- Use the "Do not disturb" or "Focus" features as often as possible.
- Enjoy boredom—don't always reach for your phone to fill the space.

Simplicity Starts before Purging

The purging part of this process is definitely the hardest, but there's a step on the path to sacred simplicity that starts long before emptying your closet. It's not just about what you're getting rid of. In order to make this lifestyle stick, it's also about buying less to begin with. I am stringent about what comes into our home. The biggest mindset shift we've had as a family is moving from a "want" mentality to a "need" mentality.

Shortly after we moved to Colorado, we said, "We really need a kayak." Then we caught ourselves and revised that to "It would be super cool to have a kayak, and we *want* a kayak, but we don't *need* a kayak." To be clear, it's fine to want things you don't need. But it's important to

Simplicity with Kids

It may seem impossible to be a minimalist with children. But this way of life is possible for everyone, even if you have kids. We have assigned chores for our children, and they get paid a small amount for each chore they do (this varies based on age and ability). We keep track of their money in a note on our phone, and when they are ready to spend it, we make the purchase for them (though there are apps for this too!). When it comes time for your child to buy something (or before you buy something for them), here are some questions to ask your kiddos:

- Are you sure you really want this?
- Is this similar to something you already have?
- You currently have $_____ [amount of money]. This purchase will require ___ percent of your money. Is there anything you'd like to save up for instead?
- Will this item stand the test of time? If it breaks within the week, will you wish you hadn't bought it, or will you still be glad you bought it?

make that distinction, because when we tell ourselves we need something, we think we have to buy that thing because it's a need. When we view something as a want and not a need, it becomes less vital that we have it. When we make fewer purchases, it reduces our carbon footprint, because nearly everything we buy uses fuel in some way, even if it's just for shipping. It also frees up our time! It takes time, effort, energy, and money to maintain so many things. And it means saving more money that could go into our savings or retirement, which means less work later!

So how do you serve as a gatekeeper for your own purchases?

Navigating Children's Gifts

It's easier to stick to simplicity when you're the only one who holds purchasing power, but there are also birthdays and holidays, not to mention grandparents and other people who want to be generous to your kiddos. These situations can be tricky, but we've found some strategies and alternatives that work for us. Here are some alternatives to traditional gifts.

- Create a wish list with links for each child for any situation when there will be presents. You can share these lists with anyone who will be giving presents. Sit down with your kids and brainstorm ideas based on their interests and hobbies.

- When you're hosting a birthday party, ask for no presents. It may be counter-cultural, but we've found that it makes our lives simpler and more enjoyable.

- Consider offering your kids a choice between having a birthday party or having an experience. We offer our kiddos the option of inviting friends over for a party or going on a small weekend trip as a family. More often than not, they choose the trip. We make lots of memories, and it doesn't cost much more than having a birthday party. We like that this gives us the opportunity to opt for experiences over things.

Generosity: The Antidote to Consumerism

When our sense of contentment is tied to what we buy and have, we can feel empty without these things. But actually, that's the point. We shouldn't be seeking contentment from things. Instead, we should be finding our contentment in Jesus.

We've found that practicing extreme generosity fills us with a kind of contentment that runs deeper than anything we might buy and gives us gratitude for the things we do have. Of course, generosity is about blessing others, but the biggest surprise is how much it blesses our lives too.

Generosity is marked by giving without expecting anything in return. While generosity is often associated with monetary gifts, it can also involve sharing our time or skills, or showing kindness and compassion to someone else. Over and over in the Bible, we are commanded to be generous: "Command them to do good, to be rich in good deeds, and to be generous and willing to share" (1 Timothy 6:18).

We can be generous with what we have, even if we don't have much, because we trust that God is our provider. Every generous act confirms our faith that he will provide. When we give to others, it helps us to be less consumed with our possessions and more concerned with the one who provides.

Our generosity allows us to be a blessing to others. In *Simple Truths*, Kent Nerburn says, "True giving is not an economic exchange; it is a generative act. It does not subtract from what we have; it multiplies the effect we can have in the world."[10] Generosity is not a one-way relationship. While we are blessing others, we are also blessed ourselves. As Jesus said, "It is more blessed to give than to receive" (Acts 20:35).

When I was in college, my pastor, Lee Mason, told us that life is like the board game Monopoly. No matter how much money you have stored up in your bank at the end of your life, the board is wiped clean and your bank is gone. It all goes back into the box. We don't often act like we believe the phrase "You can't take it with you." I want to live my life simply so I have more to give to others.

I want the simplicity of my life to amplify God's voice so I can follow his commands and live my life with the love and purpose he commands.

Simplicity Challenge

Beginner challenge: Every weekend for a month, choose one room of your house to simplify. Follow the tips in this chapter, and record your progress in a journal. At the end of the month, reflect on how it feels to have less stuff and less clutter.

Intermediate challenge: You have two options for the intermediate challenge. Give away one thing per day for a month, or do one act of generosity or kindness every day for a month. At the end of the month, reflect on how the process made you feel. Do you feel more grateful for the things you do have? Do you feel less inclined to buy new things?

Advanced challenge: Try a no-spend month—don't spend money aside from essentials such as groceries, housing, and utilities. We've done a "no-spend November" a number of times, and it helps me practice gratitude for what I already have. It takes some planning, so be sure to look ahead and see if you need to buy anything like birthday presents the month before. Another option is to go through your clothes and create a capsule wardrobe. Choose a number of items of clothing you want to stick to. Lay everything in your capsule wardrobe out together so you can ensure it all mixes and matches well to maximize your items.

CHAPTER 7

HEALTHY WORLD

You cannot get through a single day without having
an impact on the world around you.

JANE GOODALL

Just as we take care of our own homes, we should take care of our larger home. We are called to be protectors of this earth, but we often feel disconnected with our personal responsibility in keeping the earth healthy. We may wonder what difference one person can make, or maybe the problems with climate change seem too abstract to get our minds around. But the reality is, individuals can (and must!) make a difference.

I'm reminded of the scene in *Finding Nemo* where Dory, the forgetful blue tang fish, gets caught in a fisherman's net. Nemo knows just what to do. He swims into the net with thousands of other fish and says, "Dad, I know what to do! We have to tell all the fish to swim down together!" Sure enough, when they all swim in the same direction while chanting, "Keep swimming!" their combined weight breaks the arm of the fishing boat, and the fish are free! A single fish swimming down wouldn't have been able to free all the fish.

When it comes to climate change, we all have our parts to play, and we have to take action together to make an impact. And while environmental concerns may seem removed from daily life, this topic has come really close to home for our family when we can't go outside because of wildfires in Oregon that cause it to rain ash here in Denver.

The environment has become a hot-button political issue, but the truth is, we were given the charge to care for the earth from the very beginning. In the Garden of Eden, God gave the first human beings the responsibility of caring for the world he made: "The LORD God placed the man in the Garden of Eden to tend and watch over it" (Genesis 2:15, NLT).

So far in humans' history, we haven't done a very good job of fulfilling this calling. According to scientists, we are living in a new geological epoch. Remember *Jurassic Park*? The Jurassic epoch is an example of a geological epoch, which typically lasts tens of thousands to millions of years. This proposed new geological epoch is called the Anthropocene epoch, "an era dominated by indelible human-made impacts to the Earth."[1] The idea that humans have made enough of a negative impact on the planet to require a new geological epoch should serve as a wake-up call to us all.

Another wake-up call was when the Intergovernmental Panel on Climate Change released a report that essentially said we have about ten years to stop the most catastrophic levels of climate change. If we don't manage to shift emissions, they believe we'll start feeling massive effects as soon as 2030.[2]

While this topic may seem a little broader in scope than what we eat or how we move our bodies or what we allow into our homes, we can't talk about healthy, intentional living without addressing the planet we live on and our responsibility to protect it. We can't have health if we have nowhere to live. We won't have air if it's too polluted to breathe. We can't drink water if our planet is plagued by drought. All around the world, homes are being destroyed by floods, monsoons, mudslides, landslides, wildfires, tornadoes, hurricanes, tsunamis, earthquakes, melting glaciers, rising sea levels, and every other imaginable natural disaster. According to a recent study, extreme weather events fueled by climate change cost the US $165 billion in a single year.[3]

But it doesn't have to be this way. While it may seem daunting to tackle something as big as climate change, the same concept applies when we make changes in our personal lives: the small, daily habits add up and gain momentum to create large-scale transformation.

Let's take composting, for example. When organic matter ends up in a landfill, its decomposition without oxygen turns it into methane, a greenhouse gas eighty times more harmful than carbon.[4] When that organic matter is composted instead, it turns into nutrient-rich soil that can sequester carbon and prevent methane emissions.

We can't have health if we have nowhere to live. We won't have air if it's too polluted to breathe. We can't drink water if our planet is plagued by drought.

In San Francisco, composting became mandatory in 2009 with the Mandatory Recycling and Composting Ordinance, a step toward their long-term goal of having zero waste. San Francisco created the first—and largest—urban food scraps composting program. It has collected more than two million tons of organic material, which has been turned into composted soil for use at local orchards, vineyards, and farms.[5] It may not have seemed like a big deal to put one banana peel in the compost bin, but just look at the massive impact the composting program has had with everyone working together.[6]

According to the Union of Concerned Scientists, Americans release "twenty-one tons of heat-trapping carbon dioxide to the atmosphere each year." That's such a large number it's hard to wrap our minds around it. To bring that number down to earth for us, that's more carbon emission than driving a car all the way around the world at the equator![7]

Emissions in the US are four times the global average.[8] The Union of Concerned Scientists studied where most of our carbon emissions come from. Most of them fall into these five categories:

• transportation
• home heating and cooling

- home appliances
- food
- purchases

The term *personal emissions*, also referred to as a *carbon footprint*, is used to describe the total amount of greenhouse gases generated by each person's actions. Although calculations vary, the average carbon footprint for someone in the United States is somewhere around sixteen tons per year, which is one of the highest rates in the world. Across the globe, the average yearly carbon footprint is closer to four tons per person.

Our carbon footprint is directly related to rising temperatures. The Nature Conservancy suggests that the average carbon footprint needs to drop to below two tons per year per person by 2050 for the best chance at avoiding a two-degree-Celsius increase in global temperature.[9]

Think through Your Transportation

According to the Union of Concerned Scientists, transportation is by far the biggest source of personal emissions (29 percent).[10] That also makes it the biggest opportunity for improvement. When it comes to transportation, 81 percent of emissions come from motor vehicles, and 19 percent come from airplanes and other transportation. This makes the kind of car you drive more important than you might have thought.

You might assume the electric car is best for the environment, but that's not necessarily the case. That's because some electric car companies are discontinuing smaller vehicles and are instead making larger ones, which are overall less efficient. You can use the website greenercars.org to compare thousands of different vehicles. They assign a "green score" to vehicles, down to the make, model, and year. If you're curious, the top two recent winners for greenest cars are the Mini Cooper SE Hardtop two-door and the Nissan Leaf.[11]

Even if you don't want to swap your car, there are other ways to help the environment. An easy way is to keep your tires inflated. If every driver in the US kept their tires properly inflated, it would save more than a billion gallons of gas each year. Did you know that keeping your car professionally tuned up can increase your miles per gallon anywhere from 4 percent to 40 percent? Even a new air filter can boost your miles per gallon 10 percent! Getting more miles per gallon means using less gas, which results in less carbon in the atmosphere.[12]

In the US, most people drive, even when other options are available, but your commute doesn't have to involve a car. If you're lucky enough to be close to work, you could consider walking or biking. Another option is to use public transportation, such as a bus or a train. Public transportation runs whether you're on it or not, so switching can drastically reduce your personal emissions. It's true that driving takes less time than public transportation, but my friends who ride the train agree that even though it takes longer, it's a more pleasant experience. Parking is usually easier at the train station, whereas it can be a hassle downtown. They also enjoy the time to read or decompress before going in to work or going home. Another eco-friendly option is to carpool to work. On average, only 23 percent of Americans carpool to work, so there's room for improvement there.[13]

Study before You Buy

Although we may not think about our purchases having an impact on the environment, the stuff we buy accounts for 26 percent of total personal emissions. This includes everything we buy and all the services we use. Although buying habits vary from person to person, one thing holds true for almost everyone: buying used can make a huge impact. When you buy a preowned item, you're giving it a new home and preventing it from going into a landfill. You're also decreasing the demand for more things to be made.

It can be hard to get into the mentality of buying used, but once you start, it's kind of addicting. I have friends who can vouch for my Goodwill talents (I'm only kind of joking!). Here's one example. Before we left on a trip to Alaska, Owen had about six pairs of athletic shorts.

We only took long pants and long-sleeved shirts to Alaska, because even though it was August, it was still cool. When we got back, he somehow had only one pair of shorts! How is that possible? We didn't even take shorts along! I digress.

The kids started school the day after we got back, and I knew he needed some shorts in the 100-degree Denver heat. So we went to Goodwill, with the plan to stop at Target if we were unsuccessful. We walked in and immediately found two perfect pairs of shorts for him. They were $3.99 each. Cue the confetti! We went to Target afterward to get three birthday presents for three separate birthday parties that week-end, and we looked for more shorts while we were there. I was shocked to discover that a pair of shorts for my seven-year-old son cost $18 at Target. I will take those $3.99 Goodwill shorts, thank you!

My biggest tip for shopping for clothes at a thrift store is to go in knowing exactly what you're looking for. If you go in willy-nilly, look-ing at every section, it's too overwhelming. Also, keep the simplicity mindset. Just because something is on sale or inexpensive doesn't mean you need it!

Clothes are an easy category to think about buying used, but you can get almost anything pre-loved. I personally enjoy it because it means what I'm getting is less expensive, so my budget goes much further *and* it's better for the environment. Everyone wins!

Tips for Avoiding Plastic and Other Disposables

Plastics are terrible for you *and* the environment. Over 99 percent of plastics are made from chemicals sourced from planet-warming fossil fuels such as gas, oil, and coal,[14] and their creation adds toxic, climate-changing gases into the air. We've only been using plastics for the last hundred years, so it's hard to know how long it will take them to decompose, but the best estimate is hundreds of years. Used plastic ends up in the oceans, in the air, on our city streets, in wildlife, and even in our bodies in the form of microplastics.

Another reason it's important to avoid plastic is because it's hard to recycle. Some places offer recycling services for hard plastics, but multilayer plastics, such as the bags many foods come in, often go in the trash.

- Shop in-store if your grocery delivery uses plastic bags, and bring your own reusable bags. You can keep a tote bag in your purse so it's available when you go shopping.
- Buy in bulk and bring your own containers to the grocery store for items like grains, dried fruits, nuts, and dried herbs and seasonings.
- Skip bagging your produce in plastic bags—you can check out without them!
- Buy direct from farmers or buy local at a farmers market. Bring your own bags to avoid food packaging.
- Switch from paper towels to reusable rags or microfiber cloths.
- Use cloth napkins instead of paper napkins.
- Use handkerchiefs instead of disposable tissues.
- Use cloth face wipes to remove makeup instead of disposable wipes or cotton pads.
- Choose reusable plates instead of disposable ones. (If reusable isn't an option, try compostable plates.)
- Use glass Pyrex dishes instead of plastic containers for leftovers.
- Avoid plastic wrap and opt for reusable beeswax-coated fabric instead.
- Use silicone bags instead of single-use plastic bags. (We use Stasher.)
- Buy glass containers for shampoo and other shower supplies. Use product refills with recyclable components from shops such as Attitude. Another option is to switch to shampoo, conditioner, and soap bars that come packaged in recyclable cardboard boxes instead of plastic.
- Buy glass containers for cleaning supplies too. We use Branch Basics, including their glass spray bottles, and we have a subscription for their cleaner concentrate, which can be used as an all-purpose cleaner, a bathroom cleaner, and a window cleaner.
- Create a zero-waste kit that you can use on the go: a reusable silicone straw (I even have one for my favorite drink—boba tea!), cloth shopping bags, travel utensils (you can even find a spork and knife combination in the camping section), and a reusable coffee mug.
- Use a reusable water bottle (glass or lead-free steel) instead of plastic water bottles.
- Dine in at restaurants instead of getting takeout. If you're getting takeout, let the restaurant know you don't need utensils, and use your own utensils at home.
- If you have a baby, use cloth diapers. (This saved us $3,000 to $4,000 per kid! We swore by the bumGenius brand.)
- Swap disposable razors with a reusable razor so you only need to replace the blades.

Upgrade Your Heating and Cooling

Home heating and cooling is the next biggest category of personal emissions, at 17 percent. We may assume every furnace and air conditioner is generally the same, but these systems can vary widely in efficiency.

I grew up with an appreciation for heating and cooling because my dad owned a commercial HVAC company and sold huge cooling towers, which he would always point out as we were driving around Nashville.

If you have an older furnace or air-conditioning unit, you might want to consider upgrading to a more efficient model. Remember, you can save money buying used while still being energy efficient. While more efficient models are definitely an up-front investment, they require less energy to run, and you will see lower power bills.

While getting newer, more efficient furnaces and air-conditioning units is a great option, it's also important to service them regularly, regardless of what type of unit you have. Be sure your furnace and air conditioner are serviced once a year, typically right before you'll be using them for the season.

You can also use sunlight to your advantage. In the winter, open all your blinds and drapes to let in as much sun as possible. This can warm your home without costing you a penny—and with zero emissions. In the summer, use blackout shades or drapes to keep the sun's heat out of your home and keep your rooms cooler.

Another cost-effective way to keep your home cool is to add or upgrade ceiling fans. Most models allow you to control whether they're sending air down or pulling air up. You want them to send the warm air that has accumulated at the top of a room down in the winter and pull that warm air up in the summer. With a simple flick of a switch, you can make a world of difference in the felt temperature of a room.

If you have pets or you don't clean your fan blades often, be sure to check them for dust before switching the direction of your fan blades. When we moved into our home in Savannah where the previous owners had cats, there was about an inch of dust and cat hair on the fan blades. Chaz switched the direction of the blades while I was sitting on the bed directly below the fan, and cat fluff and dander started raining down on me. I am insanely allergic to cats, and this is still one of my worst memories of all time. Don't repeat the same mistakes we've made!

Another way to reduce your emissions is to simply use your heater and air conditioner less frequently, keeping the temperature of your home warmer in the summer and cooler in the winter. For both cost-saving and environmental reasons, we tend to keep our home at the far end of what's considered normal temperatures. I know I'm touching on what might be a sore point in your marriage—so many couples have different preferences when it comes to the thermostat!

So what temperature should you be aiming for? In the winter, you want to keep your thermostat as low as you can while still being comfortable, which the US Department of Energy says is typically 68 degrees. (Keep in mind, if you have a heat pump, lowering your heat too much can make it less efficient.) In the summer, you want to keep your thermostat as high as you can. I recommend that you shoot for 78 degrees.

A programmable thermostat can help you maximize your energy and cost savings. If you work away from home, you can program it to be up or down 10 degrees while you're gone. We have a smart thermostat that has an "eco mode" and gives us tips to conserve energy. You can also adjust the temperature while you're sleeping. According to the US Department of Energy, "You can save as much as 10% a year on heating and cooling by simply turning your thermostat back 7°–10°F for 8 hours a day from its normal setting."[15]

My biggest tip for adapting to colder or warmer temperatures than you're used to is to adjust your clothing! When I'm too cold, that's my sign that I need a blanket or more clothes. We like to layer in the wintertime, and we do the opposite in the summer. We're all in shorts and tank tops inside, and we manage to stay pretty comfortable.

Sealing Windows and Doors

One of the biggest energy drains in homes is leaky doors and windows. According to the Union of Concerned Scientists, "Air leaks in the average

US home may squander 15 to 25 percent of the heat our furnaces generate in winter and account for the same amount of unwanted heat our homes gain in summer. That's equivalent to leaving a window in your home wide open all the time."[16]

Not only is sealing your home better for the environment, but it will also save you money on power bills. The two strategies the Department of Energy recommends are caulking and weather-stripping. Caulking is usually used for cracks and openings for stationary components in your home (around your door and window frames). Weather-stripping is used to seal movable components such as doors and operable windows.[17] You can also hire an energy assessor to check the air tightness of your home and hire someone to professionally seal your home.

If you decide to replace your windows, look for the Energy Star label and the National Fenestration Rating Council (NFRC) label, which gives energy performance ratings. If replacing your windows is not in your budget right now, you could consider adding interior or exterior low-emissivity storm windows. These have a similar benefit to double-pane new windows but are about a third of the cost. Some states have programs that give you rebates for weatherizing your home.

Analyze Home Energy Use

While home heating and cooling systems account for 17 percent of our total emissions, other home energy use accounts for 15 percent. This includes power used for electronics and appliances.

If you own your home, you can upgrade your appliances to Energy Star appliances, which meet strict energy-efficiency specifications set by the EPA.[18] I recommend doing this each time you need to replace an appliance rather than doing an overhaul of all your appliances at once. And remember, you can get newer Energy Star appliances pre-loved!

We had an issue with our water heater recently, and when the plumber came, he asked us the last time we had it serviced. Chaz and I stared at each other blankly, then looked back at the plumber. "Um, never?" Guys, someone needs to create a list of things you're just expected to know when you buy a home! We had no idea certain appliances needed to be serviced *yearly*! Having your furnace serviced ensures that everything is working properly and is operating as efficiently as possible. You can also have your ducts cleaned (see chapter 5 for more on this). Not only does this make your home less toxic since dust collects toxins, but it also makes your furnace function more efficiently.

Did you know you can set the temperature on your water heater? The suggested energy-saving temperature is 120 degrees. For every 10 degrees you're able to lower your water heater, you can save anywhere from 3 to 5 percent on water heating costs. Plus, this lowers emissions.[19]

If your dishwasher has a quick cycle, give it a try. On our dishwasher, the normal cycle runs something like two hundred minutes, while the quick cycle is seventy minutes. The quick setting is the only one we use. That means for every dishwasher load we run, we're using less than half of the normal power.

When you do laundry, it's best to wash a full load. A cold-water cycle uses the least amount of power. Fun fact: hot water sets stains, so using cold water also helps you keep stains out of your clothes. Another tip that can save you power (and money) is to run the fifteen-minute cycle. This cycle takes about one-fourth of the time and power, and it does a great job for clothes that aren't especially dirty.

Reduce Phantom Load

The term *phantom load* (also known as vampire energy or ghost load) sounds a lot creepier than it is. It simply refers to the electricity your appliances use when they're turned off but are still plugged in. The Department of Energy says standby power accounts for 5 to 10 percent of residential energy use, and it could cost as much as one hundred dollars per year for each household.[20]

Appliances that use standby power include chargers, TVs, DVD and Blu-ray players, cable boxes, satellite TV boxes, video game consoles, desktop computers, printers, stereos, microwaves, toasters, air fryers, slow cookers, Instant Pots, coffee makers, and hair dryers. Even if

Ways to Reduce Phantom Load

- **Use a power strip with a switch.** If you use a surge-protector power strip with an on/off switch, you can plug any nearby appliances into it. When you unplug or turn off the power strip, the appliances are truly off and not using phantom power.

- **Unplug your products.** Of course, there are appliances that need to remain plugged in (like your refrigerator!). But a lot of products don't need to be plugged in all the time (like your toaster or coffee maker), and you can simply unplug them until you need them again.

- **Upgrade to Energy Star products.** Energy Star appliances use lower standby power. When you need to replace your next appliance, do some research to find an energy-efficient model.

your laptop is fully charged, if it's plugged in, it's still pulling power.[21] The older the product or appliance, the more standby power it uses (I see you, VHS player!). So prioritize unplugging devices you rarely use.

A side benefit to reducing your phantom load is that this also decreases your exposure to electromagnetic fields, or EMFs (see more about this in chapter 5). There is a lot of overlap in appliances that use phantom power and those that are high in EMFs. When you put these electronics on a power strip or unplug them when you're not using them, you're accomplishing three things: lowering emissions, reducing your EMF load, and decreasing your power bill! A triple win!

Optimize Lighting

It may seem obvious, but a great way to minimize your energy usage is to turn off your lights when you're not using them. There are likely times during the day when you can open your drapes or blinds and do fine with no lighting at all. Make it a habit to turn off the lights when you leave a room (and encourage your family members to do the same!).

I don't recommend compact fluorescent light bulbs (CFLs) because they emit high amounts of EMFs, as well as UV light. Fluorescent light bulbs also have high EMF exposure. Incandescent light bulbs don't produce EMFs, but they're not very efficient. I avoid smart light bulbs, as their connection to Wi-Fi causes them to emit carcinogenic radio frequencies.[22]

The most energy-efficient light bulbs are light-emitting diode (LED) light bulbs. They require less power to produce bright light (which means fewer emissions), they have a low operating temperature, and they basically last forever. Okay, not forever, but they last, on average, 25,000 hours. If you used them twenty-four hours a day, seven days a week, that translates to several years! As a bonus, the cost to run an LED light bulb is significantly less than it costs to use fluorescent or incandescent light bulbs.[23]

LED light bulbs are the most energy efficient, but are they the best for our health? Unfortunately not, since LED light bulbs emit a high level of EMFs. Additionally, they produce a type of blue light that suppresses the production of melatonin, which promotes sleep. I like "clean LED" light bulbs, like the ones created by SaticShield. They're called "SaticPulse," and they provide the benefits of LED light bulbs without the drawbacks of dirty electricity and EMF exposure. The downside is that they're more expensive than traditional LED light bulbs.

If clean LED light bulbs aren't in the budget, the next best option for avoiding EMFs is to use incandescent light bulbs. In terms of your pocketbook and the environment, the best compromise is traditional LEDs. Sometimes we can't have it all, and that's okay. Choose your priority in this area and commit to it.

Consider Solar Power

One way to reduce your personal emissions is to switch from generated power to solar power. Instead of using coal or natural gas to power your home, why not use the sun, which is shining on your roof anyway? Solar power for a single home saves 546 to 874 kilowatt-hours (kWh) of energy from being used by power plants each year.[24] And while this can be an investment up front, it can save you money in the long term.

In Colorado, a home that uses 100 percent solar power to cover their electrical needs saves more than a thousand dollars a year. This results in a total savings of $25,500 to $33,000 on electricity.[25] A number of states subsidize solar power, so you may be able to install a system on your roof for no more than the cost of your current power bill. (Which is how it worked for us!)

Tips for Using Less Water

I will never forget my high school biology teacher telling us that the water we currently have on our planet is the only water we'll ever have. This had a lasting impact on me. With faucets that turn on without hesitation and showers that show no sign of slowing down, it can be hard to remember that water truly is a finite resource.[26]

- Turn off the water while you scrub your hands, brush your teeth, and shave.
- Only run the dishwasher when it's full, and use the fastest cycle.
- Only run full loads of laundry, and use the fastest cycle.
- If you have a dishwasher, don't hand-wash dishes. It uses more water than the dishwasher.
- Check faucets, toilets, showerheads, hoses, and sprinklers for leaks, and fix them.
- When you need to replace your toilet, choose a dual-flush or low-flow toilet (or add a conversion kit).
- If you need to water the lawn, do so in the early morning when the sun won't evaporate the water as quickly.
- Install rain sensors on your irrigation system so it won't turn on if it has rained recently.
- Buy a rain barrel to catch rain for your lawn and garden.
- Check the water usage on your water bill to be sure there are no spikes, which could be an indicator of a leak, running toilet, or drippy faucet that could be fixed.
- Ask your local government if they will do a water audit, which is often provided for free. This provides you with an inventory of how your water is currently being used and tips for how to maximize your water efficiency, which in turn saves you money!
- Go to a car wash instead of washing your car yourself—this can save up to one hundred gallons of water.
- When it's time to replace your appliances, choose high-efficiency replacements.
- Take shorter showers (showers use five to ten gallons of water per minute).
- Install water-saving showerheads (these can reduce your water usage to three gallons per minute).
- Use native and drought-resistant plants in your landscaping.
- Put a layer of mulch around trees and plants to slow down the evaporation of moisture.

Start Composting

Composting is a great way to lower your carbon footprint. When your food scraps and organic matter are trapped in landfills, they create methane gas. Composting, on the other hand, takes your food scraps and turns them into soil, right in your backyard!

You can keep your scraps in a small metal compost container in your kitchen and then, if you have access to a yard, you can put the scraps in a big compost tumbler outside. If you're in an urban setting or don't have a yard, you could get a kitchen composter (such as the Lomi) that transforms your compost into soil while you sleep.

For me, the best part about making my own compost is completing the whole cycle and then using the compost in my own garden. As an added benefit, composting keeps your trash less stinky!

The Need for Large-Scale Change

While the role we play as individuals is critical, the solution to climate change will most certainly need to involve larger forces at play. Corporations will need to change their practices to follow environmentally friendly guidelines; entire nations will need to come together; governments will need to change laws.

Sometimes I get discouraged when I think about how daunting the problem of climate change is, and I wonder what impact my personal choices can have. But while we might feel like our actions are small, they can have significant ripple effects—especially when we have the power to vote.

I'm not advocating for a specific party here; I'm encouraging you to vote for your values. Do some research, and vote for people who are committing to practices that protect the world we've been entrusted with. In addition to voting, speak up! Let your elected officials know you care about stopping climate change and you want to see legislation that will make it happen.

When I was sixteen years old, I was lieutenant governor at Youth

Environmental Protection Policies to Petition For

There are a number of ways to contact your representatives. In the United States, the legislative branch is made up of the House of Representatives and the Senate (collectively known as Congress), and citizens have representatives in both the House and the Senate. First, you'll need to find out who your representatives are. You can find your representatives online at usa.gov/elected-officials. Find your federal officials and click on their websites. Most websites have a clear email or contact button front and center. When writing to your officials, I recommend including your full name, what city you live in, and that you are a constituent— this gets their attention![27]

If you're not sure what climate-change initiative to contact your representative about, here are some ideas:

- Find strategies to limit carbon emissions.
- Initiate a charge for carbon emissions on corporations (a carbon tax) to encourage lower emissions and to encourage a shift to more earth-friendly fuel sources. More than forty countries have already successfully implemented a carbon tax, and while the goal is long-term mitigation of rising global temperatures, even in the short term, this has decreased carbon emissions. These carbon emissions contribute to ambient (outdoor) pollution, which the World Health Organization (WHO) claims, along with household air pollution, is associated with 7 million premature deaths annually from health conditions such as heart disease and lung cancer.[28]
- Create clean energy standards, which require energy companies to get a certain percentage of their power from renewable or low-emission sources such as solar and wind.
- Advocate for international environmental agreements, like the Paris Agreement.
- Advocate for adaptation policies, which help areas affected by climate change become more adaptable to extreme weather conditions.
- Adopt policies that support regenerative agriculture, organic agriculture, and no-till practices.
- Invest in renewable energy, nuclear energy, and carbon-capture technologies.[29]
- Invest in geoengineering projects such as tree planting.
- Protect public wildlands.
- Stop offshore drilling.

Legislature in Tennessee, and we met in the actual chambers at the capitol. One thing that became clear to me then is that representatives fight for what their constituents want. Why? It's in their best interest to make their constituents happy, because their constituents are the ones who vote to expel them or keep them in power. So make your voice heard!

I realize environmental concerns may seem overwhelming, but I recommend that you think about which problem—and solution—you're most passionate about. Let your representatives know about this concern, share a strategy that could help battle climate change, and explain why it's important for the government to do something about it.

Healthy World Challenge

Beginner challenge: Try a "less plastic" month. Keep all the plastic you purchase over the next thirty days in a bag so you can increase awareness of your plastic consumption.

Intermediate challenge: Switch your plastic and single-use items to reusable alternatives. Start composting! All you need to start is a bin inside your home and a composter in your yard!

Advanced challenge: Exclusively buy pre-loved for thirty days! Shop for clothes and other goods at secondhand stores such as Goodwill, Salvation Army, ThredUp, Poshmark, Mercari, or your local thrift store.

PART THREE

Connection

CHAPTER 8

BUILDING MENTAL RESILIENCE

Happiness can be found, even in the darkest of times,
if one only remembers to turn on the light.
HARRY POTTER AND THE PRISONER OF AZKABAN

Changing one simple thought can have a massive impact, like a pebble thrown into a lake. When I was preparing to run my first cross-country race, I had been telling myself, *I can't do this.* Then a friend told me, "You've got this, Caroline! If I can do it, you can do it!" Switching my mindset to *I can do this!* meant the difference between quitting when I came to a massive hill and finishing the race.

What goes on in our minds affects nearly everything in our lives, so it's important to have a healthy view of stress, healthy methods for processing stress, positive thoughts toward ourselves and others, and confidence that we can be the hero in our own story.

The way we view the world affects nearly every aspect of our lives. So much of how we interpret what happens to us and what we expect to happen to us in the future has to do with our worldview.

You know the glasses they hand you when you walk into a 3D movie? The ones that are red on the left and blue on the right? If you look at anything besides the movie specifically made for those glasses, it looks wonky. This is also how our worldview affects us—we're looking at the world through the lens of our beliefs, as well as our past, our present, and our future. If our worldview is skewed, it can distort the way we see reality.

There's a lot going on in these noggins of ours. Almost everything we think about stems from our brains (sorry-not-sorry for the pun—I just had to!). To a large degree, our mental health is determined by what we think about, how we talk to ourselves, and how we view stress.

In recent years, we've heard the term *mental health* thrown around a lot. So, for clarity's sake, let's talk about what this really means. The Centers for Disease Control and Prevention says that mental health "includes our emotional, psychological, and social well-being. It affects how we think, feel, and act. It also helps determine how we handle stress, relate to others, and make healthy choices."[1]

According to the National Institute of Mental Health, more than one in five adults in the United States live with a mental illness (that's around 58 million people).[2] No matter where we fall on the spectrum of mental health, we all go through ups and downs. Sometimes we're thriving and feeling great, and other times we are anxious or down or overwhelmed. Our mental health is constantly changing, because the demands on us are always changing.

What Stress Does to Your Body

One of the most common assaults on our mental health is stress. We all experience stressors on a daily basis, so a critical part of embracing a healthy lifestyle is learning how to process and deal with stress.

We tend to compartmentalize when it comes to our health, assuming the mind is separate from the body and the soul. But when Jesus was asked about the most important commandment, he said, "Love the Lord your God with all your heart and with all your soul and with all your mind" (Matthew 22:37). We flourish with our whole being, and we also suffer with our whole being.

It's important to recognize the difference between stress and anxiety. Stress is typically an emotional response to an external trigger—it comes and then goes. Anxiety, on the other hand, is an emotional response without a trigger. Anxiety is typically marked by excessive worries that don't go away. When you're feeling anxious, you may not even be able to identify the source of your worries.[3] Here's what Jesus had to say about this: "Do not be anxious about your life, what you will eat or what you will drink, nor about your body, what you will put on. Is not life more than food, and the body more than clothing?" (Matthew 6:25, ESV). When we trust that a good, powerful God is taking care of us, it has a way of putting our anxiety and stress in perspective.

> Two things are important when it comes to stress: our perception of stress and how we deal with it.

The World Health Organization describes stress as "a state of worry or mental tension caused by a difficult situation. Stress is a natural human response that prompts us to address challenges and threats in our lives." The key isn't to avoid stress; it's "the way we respond to stress . . . [that] makes a big difference to our overall well-being."[4]

When we first moved from Georgia to Colorado, some of my friends came out for a reunion trip in the winter. Since we had some pregnant mamas in the group, we decided to skip the skiing and try snowshoeing instead. It was a winter wonderland—it felt like we were crunching through Narnia and Aslan might show up at any moment.

Instead, when we rounded a bend, we saw a mama moose and her baby calf about twenty feet from us. If you don't live in moose territory, I'll let you in on a little secret: moose are *large* animals. Adult females weigh between 800 and 1,300 pounds and stand about seven feet tall. Given that moose are herbivores and eat mostly plants, they are not typically aggressive. Except for a mama moose that's protecting her baby calf!

As soon as we saw the moose and her baby, we froze. We had a choice to make: Would we turn around to avoid close contact with the protective moose, or would we walk past her to get to our destination? I was adamant that we needed to turn around and not mess with mama moose, but I was outvoted. Instead, we risked our lives and snowshoed by, getting way too close for my comfort. Clearly, we survived the encounter, since I'm here to tell the tale, but this story highlights how our systems are wired for a fight-or-flight response.

When there's a perceived threat, our bodies go on high alert. From there, we choose fight (*I'm going to take this mama moose head-on*) or flight (*I'm going to run away to a safe spot*). *Fight or flight* is a shortened term, and there are actually a lot more *f*s. The full term is *fight, flight, freeze, or fawn. Freezing* refers to stopping in place, as solid as if Frozone from the *Incredibles* froze you with his icy blast! *Fawning* refers to trying to please someone to avoid conflict and is used only after one of the first three options has failed. The goal of all these responses is to avoid danger and remain calm, which can be helpful for survival.[5]

Unfortunately, the response that's intended to keep us safe from physical threats like animal attacks can pose long-term harm to our health. Our minds are powerful, and our bodies respond in the same way physiologically to a real threat and a perceived one.[6] So our stress about a tough conversation we *might* have in the future cues the same response in our bodies as a fight with a spouse that actually happened—and the same response we'd have if a bear walked into our house!

When our perceived threats are near-constant, we remain in fight-or-flight mode as our default setting. This results in chronic stress. Our stress response is intended to last for a short time and then resolve—our sympathetic nervous system should be adaptive, meaning that just minutes after facing a stressor, we are no longer in fight-or-flight mode. But if we have a delayed resolution, it could take our bodies hours to return to a non-elevated state. And if we're in a state of chronic stress, it can take months to years for our bodies to reset.

Stress affects nearly every part of our bodies and our health. That's because "intense stress over-activates the immune system, leading to the imbalance [of] inflammation."[7] Inflammation is the building block for all diseases, which means that stress can ultimately harm every system of the body. When stress is chronic, it depletes our bodies' resources and hinders their ability to heal.[8]

There are many side effects to living in a state of chronic stress. You may experience muscle tension, chronic migraines, tension headaches, or low back pain. Shallow breathing from stress can trigger pre-existing conditions such as panic attacks and asthma attacks. Since stress causes increased heart rate and higher blood pressure, chronic stress can contribute to long-term complications with the heart and blood vessels, elevating your risk for hypertension, heart attack, and stroke. Stress increases the cortisol in your body, which in turn elevates your blood sugar (this is intended to provide you with the energy to fight, if necessary). In the long term, elevated cortisol and blood sugar levels can lead to metabolic disorders such as obesity and diabetes. Stress can change the bacteria in your gut, and it affects digestion and nutrient absorption.

When the body is in a fight-or-flight state, it also stops processes that aren't essential for survival. One of the first processes to go is reproduction. That's why chronic stress can lead to decreased testosterone production, erectile dysfunction, sperm production and maturation, and impotence in men. In women, chronic stress can affect fertility, causing cycles to become irregular or stop entirely.[9] In addition, long-term stress puts you at risk for anxiety, depression, digestive problems, sleep complications, weight gain, and memory and concentration impairment.[10]

Physical Signs of Stress

Although stress may begin in our minds, it often manifests itself in our bodies. According to Yale Medicine, symptoms of chronic stress fall into four categories: cognitive, emotional, physical, and behavioral. If you're experiencing three to five of these symptoms for more than a few weeks, it could be due to chronic stress.[11]

- Aches and pains
- Insomnia or sleepiness
- Change in social behavior
- Low energy
- Unfocused or cloudy thinking
- Change in appetite
- Increased alcohol or drug use
- Change in emotional responses to others
- Emotional withdrawal

Stress Is Inevitable

Before I went to school to become a health coach, I assumed that all stress is bad and that our goal should be to get our stress down to zero. But did you know there's also a good kind of stress? Mental health professionals call this *eustress* (harmful stress is called *distress*). According to Stanford professor Robert Sapolsky, "If a stressor isn't too extreme, is only transient, and occurs in what overall feels like a benevolent environment, it's great, we love it—that's what play and stimulation are."[12] Having a stress response without a fear of impending danger can actually help you focus and get things done!

Even if we tried to escape it, stress is unavoidable. As I wrote that sentence, this thought popped in my head: *Is it really, though? What if you were in a room and had every single thing provided for you? No responsibilities, no one relying on you, no need to make money?* Then I realized that sounds like jail, and I would *definitely* be stressed in that situation. So it's not a matter of eliminating our stress. Instead, there are two things that are important when it comes to stress: our perception of stress and how we deal with it.

How We Perceive Stress

My husband, Chaz, is a big believer in instilling grit in our children—more formally known as resiliency. "Individuals who have experienced a moderate amount of adversity in the past exhibit more resilience to recent adversity, suggesting that previous experiences with stress may help individuals cope with current stress."[13]

One study indicates that stress alone isn't what negatively affects health. Rather, it's about the way that stress is viewed. Individuals who perceived high levels of stress increased the risk of premature death by 43 percent.[14] Other studies have shown that having negative or pessimistic expectations of life events is predictive of poor physical and mental health and increased use of the health care system.[15] The bottom line is that the way we view our circumstances greatly impacts our health, as well as our life expectancy!

I can personally attest to the power of taking a level of ownership over our own health. When I was struggling with digestive issues as a child, I very much felt like a victim of my circumstances. Part of the reason I started my company, Olive You Whole, was because I felt empowered by the idea that God has given us the tools we need to be healthy—in mind, body, and soul. I'm a huge believer that the body wants to heal, and that belief has propelled me to find healing for myself and others.

We will always have stress. But we don't have to let that stress us out!

How We Deal with Stress

Since stress is here to stay, we have to learn how to deal with it. The incredible thing about our brains is that they are adaptable. So the same brains that get stuck in fight-or-flight mode can also be used to get us out again. Fortunately, there are proven strategies that can help us decrease the amount of negative stress we feel.

Strategies to Get out of Fight-or-Flight Mode

- Praying or meditating
- Practicing gratitude
- Journaling
- Eating sufficient protein and eating clean foods
- Doing breathing exercises
- Moving your body
- Getting consistent sleep (ideally eight hours a night)
- Having a social support network
- Eliminating unnecessary stressors when possible
- Spending time in nature
- Exposing your eyes to sunlight, especially in the morning
- Having a sense of humor
- Prioritizing your to-do list and choosing the three most-necessary tasks each day
- Taking breaks from the news and social media
- Taking a bath
- Getting a massage
- Participating in hobbies you enjoy
- Trying new activities
- Diffusing essential oils in your home

One way to handle stress more effectively is to exercise. We already talked about how beneficial exercise is for our bodies, but it's also a powerful way to keep our minds healthy. "One of the most devastating consequences of chronic stress is that it damages stress's off switch. This makes the body stress resistant, allowing cortisol to rise to uncontrollably

How to Practice Box Breathing

1. Slowly take a deep breath for four counts.
2. Hold it for four counts.
3. Exhale for four counts.
4. Hold it for four counts.
5. Repeat.

high levels that damage the body and mind." Exercise is powerful because it releases a protein that counteracts the toxic effects of high stress.[16]

Another helpful tool in dealing with stress is intentional breathing. When we're experiencing stress, we tend to hold our breath or take shallow breaths. Breath work involves slowing down our breathing as we inhale and exhale deeply. This activates our parasympathetic nervous system, helping restore a sense of calm. Countless studies have shown the benefits of breathing exercises, including improvement in categories such as depression, stress, mental health, positive affect, mindfulness, and social connectedness.[17]

There are many different types of breathing exercises you can do. When I'm feeling signs of stress, my favorite technique is called "box breathing." Navy SEALs, who are often in high-stress, high-pressure environments, use box breathing to remain calm.[18]

Taking Your Thoughts Captive

A big part of mental health comes down to something that sounds simple: our thoughts. Mastering our thoughts can benefit every part of our lives. But we all know just how unruly and uncontrollable our thoughts can be.

The first step in controlling any kind of negative thought is to take inventory of your thoughts. Are you trash-talking yourself? Are you consumed by judgmental thoughts about those around you? Are you obsessing over what someone did to you? These kinds of thoughts may be so deeply ingrained that you don't even realize they're there.

After you take inventory of your thoughts, take them captive. In 2 Corinthians 10:5, Paul tells us to "take every thought captive to obey

Christ" (ESV). We don't want to allow these thoughts to live rent-free in our brains.

But how do we get rid of them? Once we recognize these thoughts, we replace them with the truth. For example, if you're in a coffee shop and someone walks in and you find yourself thinking, *Wow, that top looks terrible on her*, stop yourself. Apologize to her silently. Then remind yourself that she is made in the image of God, just like you are.

Thousands of thoughts run through our minds in a day, and the way we think can change how we feel about ourselves, how we think about others, and ultimately how we talk to and treat others. As we transform our thoughts, we become more like Jesus. Romans 12:2 says, "Do not be conformed to this world, but be transformed by the renewal of your mind, that by testing you may discern what is the will of God, what is good and acceptable and perfect" (ESV). When our minds are transformed, we gain the freedom and peace he offers.

Quieting Your Inner Critic

Let's talk about how we talk to ourselves. When our self-talk is negative, it's often referred to as our "inner critic." Have you ever taken inventory of the thoughts inside your head and monitored the way you talk to yourself? I'm not talking about passing thoughts like *Oh, I need to add butter to my grocery list*, but the voice in your head that is either cheering you on or passing judgment on your worth.

The inner critic may tell you that you look fat when you look in

Using Positive Affirmations

If you consistently tell yourself that you're terrible at getting things done, you start to believe it. But the flip side is also true. Our brains want to be right—we get a dopamine rush when we accurately predict an outcome or get something right. So when we tell ourselves, *I'm productive!* we will act differently to prove ourselves right.

Positive affirmations can be anything you tell yourself! Just fill in the blank: "I am _____." Some examples include "I am enough," "I am joyful," "I am brave," or "I am getting better every day." If you would prefer to combine positive affirmations with words God has spoken over you, some examples include "I am known" (see Psalm 139:1-4), "I am beloved" (see Ephesians 2:4-5), "I am forgiven" (see Ephesians 1:7), and "I am healed" (see Isaiah 53:5).

the mirror while trying on clothes. Maybe she reminds you that you're not brave enough to speak up at a team meeting. Maybe she tells you that you'll never amount to anything or that you'll never be loved. If the voice of this inner critic is frequent and loud in your brain, it's enough to start making you believe things about yourself that simply aren't true.

There's another option besides the inner critic, and it's what I've heard described as the "inner best friend."[19] When we take inventory of our thoughts, we can ask ourselves, *Would I talk to my best friend that way?* If the answer is no, then it's time to change the tone of our self-talk to align with the way we'd talk to a friend.

Putting a Check on Judgment

We are surrounded by impossibly high standards—standards that have been placed on us without our consent. Thanks to a constant stream of media, we're given narrow guidelines about what beauty looks like, what we should wear, how much we should weigh, how our home should be decorated, what kind of house we should live in, where we should go on vacation, and how we should raise our children. When we have a judgmental thought about someone else, what we're really doing is telling ourselves that they're not following the "rules" and we're doing it better. Many times when we judge someone, it's really not about them; it's about wanting to feel better about ourselves.

Jesus said, "Do not judge, and you will not be judged. Do not condemn, and you will not be condemned. Forgive, and you will be forgiven. Give, and it will be given to you. A good measure, pressed down, shaken together and running over, will be poured into your lap. For with the measure you use, it will be measured to you" (Luke 6:37-38). I definitely don't want to be measured by my own harsh judgments. That's why it's my goal to switch my judgmental thoughts with truth. When I'm tempted to look down on someone else, I try to ask myself, *What would Jesus see in this person?*

The more we judge others, the more we judge ourselves too. Our eyes and brains can get in the negative habit of looking for the bad instead of the good—in ourselves and others. We don't need that kind of negativity in our lives. That's why this retraining of the brain to find and think about the good can be so beneficial for our mental health.

Letting Go of What Other People Think

Chaz is an Enneagram 9, also known as "the peacemaker" or "the mediator." He is the definition of "go with the flow." This mentality permeates everything in his life, and he truly doesn't care what other people think of him. He hasn't had social media since he took his first board exam for medical school twelve years ago.

To be clear, that is not my tendency at all! There's a certain pressure that comes from living your life on social media. But I try to learn from Chaz's mentality (and he reminds me often!). He lives for God, himself, and his family, and he doesn't worry too much about getting the approval of anyone else.

In the book *The Courage to Be Disliked*, Ichiro Kishimi and Fumitake Koga say that being disliked is "proof that you are exercising your freedom and living in freedom, and a sign that you are living in accordance with your own principles."[20] Always considering what other people will think of your choices causes unnecessary stress and anxiety. Jesus was only concerned about pleasing his Father: "I seek not to please myself but him who sent me" (John 5:30). We, too, should be living for God's approval, not the approval of others.

When we get to the end of our lives, we don't want to regret worrying about what other people thought of us. According to hospice nurse and *New York Times* bestselling author Hadley Vlahos, one of people's top three life regrets is not doing something because of what someone else would think. One patient told her, "I didn't do what I wanted to do because I was so afraid of what Betty down the street thought of me, and you know what? Betty down the street is dead. She can't think anything, and I didn't get to do what I wanted to do!"[21] There is freedom that comes with letting go of what other people think of you!

Embracing Forgiveness

You may not have thought about it in these terms, but forgiveness is a wellness issue. In a study of almost five thousand people in high-conflict countries, participants completed a forgiveness intervention workbook. Doing so resulted in an increased ability to forgive, a reduction in depression and anxiety, and increased flourishing, including happiness, life satisfaction, mental and physical health, meaning, purpose, and social relationships.[22]

When we're talking about forgiveness, we have to start with the greatest example of forgiveness of all time: Jesus died on the cross and gave his life as a sacrifice to save us from our sins. That means the worst things anyone has ever done can be forgiven. In the whole world. For all time. Not a single thing is "too bad" to receive his love and forgiveness. Ephesians 4:32 says, "Forgive one another as quickly and thoroughly as God in Christ forgave you" (MSG). God didn't present forgiveness to us as an option; it's a command. It's also a gift. You might assume forgiveness is a gift to the person you're forgiving. But in reality, when you forgive someone for the hurt they've caused, you are the one who receives a gift—the gift of peace.

Let me clarify something here: forgiveness is *not* saying, "What you did is okay" or "The thing you did to hurt me is excusable." Absolutely not. Forgiveness is also not about being a doormat and letting people walk all over you. You still need to set boundaries and stand firm about how you will and will not be treated. But forgiveness allows you to move past the hurt that was done to you and live a life of flourishing.

We might feel like holding on to a grudge gives us power over the person who has hurt us. But in my experience, your offender is not likely awake at night, feeling guilty over what they've done. They don't wake up every morning with bated breath, hoping that today is the day you'll forgive them. Truthfully, your lack of forgiveness isn't punishing anyone other than *you*.

So instead of thinking of forgiveness as letting someone else off the hook, think of it as setting yourself free! When you forgive someone, you are trading your resentment and bitterness for your own sense of peace.

But *how* do we forgive someone? Everett Worthington, a licensed clinical psychologist and professor emeritus at Virginia Commonwealth University and researcher on forgiveness, uses the acronym REACH to explain the process for forgiveness: recall the hurt, empathize, altruistic gift, commit, hold on to forgiveness. You remember what happened, you remember both how you felt and how the other person could have been feeling, you give forgiveness without expecting anything in return, you choose forgiveness, and you hold on and remember that you truly did forgive.[23]

Eva Kor was a Hungarian Jew who survived imprisonment in an Auschwitz concentration camp. In 2015, at the age of eighty-one, Eva attended the trial of a man named Oskar Groening, a former German SS sergeant who later served time in jail for being complicit in the murder of 300,000 people.[24] When she came face-to-face with her captor, she didn't rail at him or try to get revenge. Instead, she hugged him and publicly forgave him.[25]

As you can imagine, many people pushed back at her willingness to forgive someone who was culpable in one of the darkest moments in world history. Even Eva's husband, Michael, said he would never follow in his wife's footsteps. But Eva said her forgiveness was "not because they deserve it, but because I deserve it."[26] She has said since, "Why survive if all you want to be is sad, angry, and hurting? That is so foreign to who I am. I don't understand why the world is so much more willing to accept lashing out in anger than embracing friendship and humanity."[27]

If Eva can forgive her captor, and if Jesus can forgive me, then I can forgive anyone.

Becoming a Hero in Your Own Story

How do you see yourself in the story that's playing out right in front of you? According to your view of the world, does life just happen to you—the good and the bad? Do you assume your circumstances are

When to Seek Professional Help

I don't think anyone can go through life with zero trauma. According to *Psychology Today*, 90 percent of adults in the United States have experienced a traumatic event at some point.[28] This definition of trauma rings true for me: "Trauma is anything that happens too much too fast." Traumatic events can be anything from a car accident to sexual assault to a natural disaster. This explains why one person may deem a certain experience traumatic when another person doesn't. In other words, trauma is personal and subjective.

Trauma is a leading factor in chronic stress, and when left unresolved, it can lead to harmful behaviors as we attempt to numb the pain. Unresolved trauma can also lead to PTSD (post-traumatic stress disorder), anxiety, and depression.

If you've been through a traumatic event and you've never been to therapy, please consider seeking professional help. Trauma can affect every aspect of your life, and working through your emotions with a professional can allow you to push through and heal from your past. Please see the list of mental help resources in appendix 2.

unavoidable and not connected to your choices? Maybe you feel like you're more of a recipient of life than a protagonist who is calling the shots. You may feel like you can't change what's going to happen, so why try? Or do you see yourself as a cocreator in your life? You feel confident that if there's something you want, you can make it happen. If something isn't working, you can tweak it until it fits your vision and goals.

The first worldview expresses a victim mentality. Donald Miller describes this in his book *Hero on a Mission*: "The victim is the character who feels they have no way out."[29] When you have a victim mentality, you feel helpless, like there's nothing you can do to escape your situation—possibly because you've had a traumatic situation in your past that was unavoidable. When someone thinks of themselves as forever the victim, they are unable to see a path forward. They regularly feel on edge, waiting for the next shoe to drop.

Someone with this mindset might feel frustrated that the world is against them—hopeless, hurt by their belief that their loved ones don't care, and resentful of happy people. A victim mentality is harmful to mental health because these feelings can lead to angry outbursts, loneliness, isolation, and depression.[30]

If this sounds like the spot you find yourself in, there is good news: you don't have to remain stuck there. The solution to a victim mindset is to realize that you can change your circumstances. When you realize that you have agency over your actions and that those actions can change the trajectory of your life, you can be released from a victim mindset.

Instead of being a victim of your circumstances, you can play the hero. *You* are the protagonist in your own story. Donald Miller describes the hero as "the character who faces their challenges and transforms."[31] As the hero, you make choices. Sometimes they're good and sometimes they're not, but you take responsibility for them. You know your choices are pointing you toward a certain kind of life. You're not just a recipient of life, but an active agent.

At this point you may be thinking, *But I'm not in control—God is!* How does this idea of being a hero mesh with our faith?

Here's the key: we are cocreators with God. Basically the entire Bible revolves around God cocreating with humans, starting from the very beginning: "The LORD God took the man and put him in the Garden of Eden to work it and take care of it" (Genesis 2:15). Pope Francis expounds upon this idea of cocreation: "'Tilling' refers to cultivating, ploughing or working, while 'keeping' means caring, protecting, overseeing and preserving. This implies a relationship of mutual responsibility between human beings and nature."[32] God gave Noah the blueprints for the ark, and Noah followed his command and built it. Moses was given instructions to create the Tabernacle, where God would dwell.

This idea of you being in the driver's seat of your life may seem like a big shift for you. Any time you change your worldview, it can be disorienting, like you've been wearing the wrong glasses and you finally get glasses with the right prescription. Even though the new glasses are correct, it can take some time for your eyes to adjust. But once you adjust, you'll find that you see the world around you much more clearly.

Mental Health Challenge

Beginner challenge: No matter where you are on your mental health journey, a good step is to start a gratitude journal. Every day for a month, write down at least one thing you're grateful for. At the end of the month, evaluate how being grateful daily impacted your overall mood, and continue to monitor to see if it also had lasting effects. Another option is to write in a journal each night and dump all your anxieties in it. I find that once I write down what I'm worried about, my concerns seem much smaller. Relieving your anxieties before bed improves your mental health and helps you sleep better!

Intermediate challenge: Take a walk every day for a month. Getting sun, especially in the morning, increases the infrared light that comes through your eyes, gives you a boost of vitamin D, regulates your circadian rhythms, and improves your mood. Spending time outdoors has so many benefits, including boosting your immune system.

Advanced challenge: Practice neuroplasticity by learning a new skill for a month. Don't worry about whether you're good at this activity—find something you enjoy doing just for fun. It could be learning to code, playing a new instrument, gardening, learning a new language, or woodworking, to name a few examples. This is a great way to stretch your brain and improve your mental health. Another option is to practice creativity each day for a month. Being creative sparks joy, happiness, and fulfillment.

CHAPTER 9

FINDING—AND BEING—
A GOOD FRIEND

*A day without a friend is like a pot without
a single drop of honey left inside.*

WINNIE THE POOH

I thought I was the most extroverted person on the planet . . . until my daughter, Ella Rae, came along. When she was in preschool, we used to go to Chick-fil-A on Fridays since she didn't have school that day. She would play in the play area for about an hour, and when we left, she would be *sobbing* about leaving her "best friend, Harper," whom she had known for . . . forty-five minutes.

As an Enneagram 7 and ENFJ on Myers-Briggs, I am a huge fan of friendship. I cherish my friends, strive to keep the relationships strong, and prioritize finding community.

Not that this has always been easy. When Chaz was in medical school, we moved a lot. But those moves taught me how to intentionally seek out community. As a young married couple in Savannah, Georgia, we immediately found a church. We loved the first place we tried—it was a start-up church with not many people, most of whom were young couples or families. Our first Sunday was in early July, and our future besties, Ben and Katie, invited us to a Fourth of July cookout. We loved hanging out with them (and everyone else from the church) so much that when they invited us to be in their small group, it was an easy yes!

I know that not everyone finds connection so quickly. Some people take time to build community while others connect immediately; some people need a big group of friends while others prefer to go deep with just a few people. Regardless of how introverted or extroverted you are and how social or reserved you are, we *all* need community.

I believe we were made for connection. In the beginning, God said, "It is not good for the man to be alone. I will make a helper suitable for him" (Genesis 2:18). God created us for relationships, and his very nature is a model of relationship for us, in the form of the Trinity (God, Jesus, and the Holy Spirit).

Benefits of Having Friends

- Increases your sense of belonging and purpose
- Boosts your happiness and reduces your stress
- Improves your self-confidence and self-worth
- Helps you cope with trauma, such as divorce, serious illness, job loss, or the death of a loved one
- Encourages you to change or avoid unhealthy lifestyle habits, such as excessive drinking or lack of exercise[1]

In this world of greater globalization, we are somehow more connected than ever and, at the same time, increasingly lonely. It seems like it should be easy to make and keep friends with people literally at our fingertips, but both research and experience tell us that's simply not the case.

We're lonelier than ever, which means we're also less healthy, happy, and mentally strong. If we want to live purposeful, meaningful lives, we need to be intentional about forming, maintaining, and prioritizing friendships.

A Surprising Requirement for Wellness

While you might not automatically think of friendship as a wellness topic, it is absolutely critical for our health! The book *The Blue Zones* explores different geographical areas around the world with the highest concentration of centenarians.[2] A crucial component of all these communities is friendship. According to Harvard Medical School, "Dozens of studies have shown that people who have satisfying relationships with family, friends, and their community are happier, have fewer health problems, and live longer."[3]

Believe it or not, friendship decreases your mortality rate. In a study of Alameda County, California, residents, "the age-adjusted relative risks for those most isolated when compared to those with the most social contacts were 2.3 for men and 2.8 for women."[4] That means that women with strong ties were three times less likely to die!

Loneliness is a wellness issue, and friendship is the solution.

The bottom line is that loneliness is a wellness issue, and friendship is the solution.

What Makes a Good Friend?

Just as you aren't perfect, you'll never find a perfect friend. But there are some general guidelines to look for in a friend (this is the way you want to treat your friends too!). A genuine friend accepts you and loves you for who you are, not who they wish you were or who they think you should be. They are open to change and are full of curiosity, not judgment. At the core, they're people you really enjoy being around. You don't have to share the same exact values as your friends, but you need friends who live with integrity, meaning they know their values and live in alignment with them.

You also need to be able to trust your friends. Trust comes from honesty, which means your friends tell you the truth, even when it's hard to hear. They hold you accountable and call you to the best version of yourself. They are dependable and keep their word, including showing up for appointments you've made together. Good friends truly listen to you. They empathize with your emotions—they can laugh with you and cry with you. They are supportive of you and cheer on your successes. They are loyal even when times are tough.

How Many Friends Do You Need?

Anthropologists have theorized that humans can only maintain about 150 relationships. Your inner circle is typically made up of around five people—these are your closest relationships, likely your immediate family. This is followed by a circle of 15 people who are your good friends, then a circle of 50 friends, 150 meaningful contacts, 500 acquaintances, and 1,500 people you recognize.[5]

I used to think more was better when it came to friendships. I felt like I had endless capacity for relationships, and any stranger could be my next best friend! As I've gotten older, though, I've started to realize the value of deep over wide. I now see the value of having a handful of friends who know just about everything about me rather than having a huge group of friends who know very little. It feels like a more meaningful and rewarding investment.

Grab a journal or a piece of paper and take a moment to reflect on your friendships.[6] Who are the five or so people in your inner circle? Who are your fifteen or so close friends? How do you feel about the number of friends in this category? If you have a lot more than fifteen, you may not be able to go as deep or be as vulnerable with them. It's possible some of the people you've put in the "close friends" category are actually just friends, not close friends. If you have a lot fewer than fifteen friends, it may be time to stretch yourself and enter into more close relationships that will benefit you emotionally, mentally, physically, and spiritually. If you hold yourself back, you're missing key opportunities to grow—and to help others grow too.

How Do You Make New Friends?

Whether you find yourself in a situation of having many surface-level friends or not pursuing enough friendships, we can all benefit from opening ourselves to new relationships. The key ingredient to creating new friendships is . . . time! According to a study out of the University of Kansas, it takes fifty hours to go from acquaintance to casual friend, ninety hours to get to good friend status, and two hundred hours to view someone as your close friend.[7]

Considering how little time we tend to set aside for rest, relaxation, and hanging out, that is a lot of time. It's a big investment—and it can be a daunting one. But since we need friendships and community for our physical, emotional, and spiritual health, it's imperative that we put in the work of forging friendships.

Okay, so we know friendship is important. But how do we go about making new friends? While children tend to make connections naturally, it seems harder as we get older. If you're wondering where to begin, remember that like most of the topics we've discussed in this book, it starts with small steps!

For starters, you can look around for people you have things in common with. Friendships are often forged around similarities. You could find someone with shared interests or hobbies. You could find someone the same age or life stage (single, newly married, mom of young kiddos, empty nesters). Or maybe you share a space—you might be neighbors, coworkers, or parents of kids on the same soccer team.

We've moved many times over the last ten years, so I know what it's like to have to start over and be in desperate need of friends. One of the best strategies I've found to build relationships is to get plugged in at a church. Whenever we move, we look for a new church, and when we find one that feels like a good fit, we waste zero time joining a small group. You might be able to meet people on Sunday mornings, but small groups are where you can go deeper.

If church isn't your thing, maybe there's a group you could join. Think of your hobbies, and then start researching groups of like-minded people. If you're having trouble finding something, utilize Facebook groups. You can create a post to find other people who are interested in your hobby. For example: "Hey, everyone! I'm a thirty-five-year-old mom of two. I want to start going on hikes midday when my kids are at school. Would anyone want to be part of a hiking group with me? Hikes will be within a thirty-minute drive of Denver, and I envision that the total time would be about three hours, once a month. Comment below if you're interested, and I'm happy to start a group text to arrange details."

If it sounds too daunting to reach out to people you don't know, look around you! No doubt there are potential friends you come into contact with as a regular part of your day. As you interact with the acquaintances around you, start paying closer attention. If anyone sticks out as a potential friend, ask them to get coffee. Chances are, they're as much in need of a friend as you are!

We moved into our home in December 2019, just a few months before the pandemic hit. By the time March rolled around and we were settled in and ready to create our community, it wasn't exactly a great time to say, "Hey, stranger, would y'all want to come over for dinner?" But I was feeling lonely in my new neighborhood, and I knew I had to do something to create the community I longed for.

One day when I was outside, I saw a family going on a midday walk. The kids looked like they were around the same age as our kids, so I decided to introduce myself. I immediately asked the mother, Alissa, for her phone number.

This family ended up being a godsend for us. They were people of faith, we all liked each other, and our kids got along! They were our quarantine buddies, and since we met, we've done Bible studies together, hosted movie nights, watched each other's kids, and gone on road trips together. Working up the courage to initiate a friendship can be hard—but it's also worth the risk!

There are times when a relationship doesn't organically go deeper, and you may need to get vulnerable to take things to the next level. It can be as simple as saying to a potential friend, "I'm really in need of some deep, intentional, Christ-honoring friendships. I'd love if we could meet once a week to deepen our friendship. Is that something you'd be interested in?" I live my life by the mantra from Brené Brown: "Clear is kind."[8] When we spell out our desires and expectations, the relationship is much more likely to go the way we hope it will.

How Do You Prioritize Friendships?

Even when we recognize the value of friendships, there are so many reasons they can get pushed to the back burner. Maybe your schedule is busy, your friend moved away, you're in a new city, you don't want to start over with new friendships, or you feel like you have enough friends on social media.

According to a study published in the *Journal of Neuroscience*, face-to-face friendships are important, because our brains are stimulated differently in in-person interactions compared to online exchanges.[9] Real-life relationships yield stronger and faster connections. I know this is true for me—I feel much more connected to someone after getting coffee or going for a walk than if we catch up on the phone (though this is still important, especially in long-distance relationships).

With so many obstacles, how do you make in-person friendships a priority? For me, this requires intentional scheduling. I know—it seems like friendships should be laid back and go-with-the-flow, but with our minute-by-minute schedules, we have to *make* time for relationships.

My friend and friendship expert Bailey Hurley sets aside one night every week as friend night. She and her husband switch off who gets to hang out with friends that night and who stays home to watch the kids. That requires some serious prioritization, but their souls are filled up because of it.

Look over your list of fifteen close friends. Now think about the last time you spent quality time with them. Do you have a regularly scheduled time to get together, or do you just wait for something to happen? Do you tend to initiate gatherings, or do you wait for someone else to do it?

In my experience, adult friendships require intentionality—they don't just happen. I recommend setting aside time weekly or monthly to be with life-giving friends. You might want to get together for coffee, dinner, or a walk. Or invite them to join you in a hobby or creative outlet. It's less important *what* you do and more important that you're consistently investing in deep friendships.

How Do You Keep Lifelong Friends?

While it's important to have in-person relationships, it's also beneficial to hold on to relationships when you and your friend no longer live in the same place. The rules for local friends apply to friends who live far away. Even if you can't get together every week, you need time together and regular connection. When you're no longer in the same city, this might look like texts, phone calls, voice memos, Facetime chats, or trips to visit each other. You can also use apps like Voxer for voice messaging or Marco Polo for video messaging.

I've found that scheduling a time to chat works better than calling on the fly, though that can work too. If you have a friend you really loved from your past who you haven't talked to in a long time, it's never too late! Ask if they would like to catch up. You can tell them you've missed them and see if they want to make your conversations a regular thing. I've found recently that sending short voice memos back and forth is a great way for me to keep up with people, because it allows my friends and me to send updates whenever we have a few minutes. It's more personal than a text, and you can cover a lot more ground in just a few minutes.

With friends I talk to or see less frequently, I find that it helps to take notes. I know, that might sound silly, but my brain can't hold on to all the information, especially if it's not information I need readily available. After a phone call, I jot down some notes on what we talked about so I can follow up the next time we talk. Keeping notes might also prompt you to pray for your friend or to check on her if you know an important date or event is coming up. You can take notes in the "notes" section of that person's contact or in your phone's notes app.

How Do You Deal with Conflict in a Friendship?

Creating and maintaining friendships can be life giving. But as we've all experienced at some point, relationships can go south. And while Jesus offers forgiveness and reconciliation, there are times when we need to

Red Flags to Watch for in a Friendship

- Someone who breaks your trust. It's hard to build an authentic relationship with someone who lies, cheats, steals, or spreads rumors.
- Someone who is overly competitive with you or unnecessarily points out your similarities and differences.
- Someone who puts you down or makes fun of you.
- Someone who gossips about others around you. If they're gossiping about someone else, they're gossiping about you too!
- Someone who bashes their spouse to you. We all need friends we can talk honestly with about struggles and frustrations. But if your friend is constantly denigrating their spouse, that's a sign to watch for.
- Someone who constantly one-ups you.
- Someone who has a victim mentality—they're stuck in a negative spiral and they refuse to get out of it. You can try to encourage someone in this spot, but if they're not open to feedback, they will end up dragging you down.
- Someone who sucks all your energy. If you find that you feel worse instead of better after spending time with them, it's probably a sign that this isn't a healthy connection for you.
- Someone who doesn't listen well or consistently cuts you off.
- Someone who always expects you to keep up the friendship and make the plans.
- Someone who doesn't prioritize the friendship.
- Someone who constantly cancels plans or doesn't show up when you're supposed to meet.
- Someone who is a bad influence or doesn't respect your values. They live in a way that's contrary to the way you want to live.
- Someone who isn't open to feedback or change.

step back from an unhealthy relationship. It's helpful to recognize warning signs as you enter friendships so you can avoid potentially harmful relationships or get a relationship back on track before unhealthy patterns are set.

None of us are perfect, and we all make mistakes. It's how we handle those mistakes that's important. If you have a friend who exhibits one or more red flags, it's important to talk to them. Tell them what you've noticed and how that makes you feel, and ask what they think about what you've shared. Emotionally healthy friends won't get defensive. They'll listen and be genuinely disappointed that they hurt you, and they'll apologize. While it can take time to get out of harmful habits, it's crucial that they're committed to rectifying the problem.

When Do You Need a Friendship Breakup?

What if your friend can't—or won't—change? How do you know when it's time for a friendship breakup?

Unless an offense is very deep, a one-time slipup shouldn't signal the end of the relationship. In my opinion, a friendship needs to end if an offense is brought to a friend's attention and discussed but continues to be a harmful pattern.

The biggest red flag for me is when I realize I'm not excited to respond to a text or call from someone or schedule a meetup with them. That's a sign that there's something about this relationship that is not life giving. This prompts me to dig deeper and see what's going on under the surface. The relationship may still be redeemable, but it's time for some self-reflection and a conversation.

What's the Difference between Friendship and Community?

Friends are critical to a healthy life, but so is community—and they aren't quite the same thing. Community is a feeling of fellowship within a group of people, often as a result of shared attitudes, interests, values, and goals. I have one-on-one friends who aren't necessarily part of a larger community. These friendships are dear to me and serve an important purpose, but it's also important to have a group of people to do life with. They know when you're going in for surgery, and they plan a meal train for you. They know when your teenager is struggling. They know when you need a hug or a walk. They know when you're having a rough day and bring you your favorite coffee drink. These are the people who are there for you day in and day out, through thick and thin.

My family has formed the strongest bonds of community through our churches. There is a rhythm to church that fosters community: church on Sunday, lunch afterward, small group during the week, maybe a hangout on the weekend. As with friendships, time and frequency are necessary to foster true community.

We were made for this kind of relational network that knits our lives together with those around us. Romans 12 says that our community as believers is like a body, and each of us has an important part to play. I think of it as a village mindset, where we live alongside each other, speak into each other's struggles, and actively participate in one another's lives.

Recently we were packing up after church and my friend (and pastor) Megan looked over at my daughter and said, "Ella Rae! Get over here—it's time to go to lunch!" And I thought, *Yes, I want more people in my life who feel comfortable giving my kids direction, guidance, and advice, in big and small ways.* I want people who know the good, the bad, and the ugly, and who know how to support me in those moments.

If you don't have community, build it yourself. Trust me, people love community. If you build it, they will come.

Friendship Challenge

Beginner challenge: Make a new friend! This friend could be an acquaintance you've always wanted to get to know better, or it could be someone brand new! Making even one new friend gives you the encouragement you need to make more friends.

Intermediate challenge: Consider your community. Do you have a village—a group of people you can turn to when you need support? If not, consider who could be part of your community and take steps to solidify these relationships for thirty days. Maybe it's your neighbors. Maybe it's a small group through church. Community is vital, and creating it often requires a conscious choice.

Advanced challenge: Take an inventory of your relationships. List as many people as you can think of—immediate family, extended family, friends, and acquaintances. From there, categorize the people on your list into where they currently fit: closest friends, good friends, circle of friends, and acquaintances. If you are looking to make new friends, your challenge is to choose one person from your list to focus on for thirty days, and commit to going deeper in that relationship by reaching out to them weekly. While the goal is an in-person meetup each week, you can also start with a weekly text or phone call. At the end of thirty days, take stock. Have you developed a deeper friendship that is life giving to both of you? You can use this same process to create stronger friendships. If you have many friends (perhaps your circle of fifteen is more like fifty), your challenge is to go from wider to deeper. The number of people you choose to focus on is up to you—you can start with just one or up to five. You might want to start with your best friend, or you could choose an acquaintance you'd like to get to know better. The goal is to invest intentional time with this person that goes beyond a typical check-in and get to know them in a deeper way. It's important to note here that you're not neglecting your other friends; you're just concentrating specifically on the person or people you've chosen.

CHAPTER 10

HARMONY AT HOME

If we love . . .we will try to do something. First in our own home.

MOTHER TERESA

Our inner circle is made up of our core relationships—the people who influence us most and who we influence most. They're the people we spend the most time with, the people we laugh with, the people who sharpen us, the people we eat with, the people who drive us crazy, the people we live out faith and homework and budgets with. If you're married with kids at home, that's likely your husband and children. If not, God has other ways of putting together people who are like family. For the sake of simplicity, this chapter talks about how to cultivate intentional relationships in the context of marriage and parenting, but the principles apply to other relationships in your inner circle as well. I'm a firm believer that chosen family is family too. Even Jesus said, "Whoever does the will of my Father in heaven is my brother and sister and mother" (Matthew 12:50).

The Bible has a lot to say about our most intimate relationships—in fact, God has described his relationship with us as a marriage, and one of the most common metaphors he uses to describe himself is as our heavenly Father. One of the first stories in the Bible is about Adam and Eve, which shows God's divine intent for companionship and kinship. One of the Ten Commandments is to honor your father and mother (something we remind our kiddos of often!).

Get to Know Yourself

Early in life, I became a big personality-test nerd, because I needed to both understand how I ticked and how other people were different than I was. I think it's so beneficial to take personality tests and get to know yourself—not only so you can know your strengths and what you have to offer, but also so you can discover your blind spots and how to check them. Knowing more about yourself isn't just for you—this knowledge helps your interactions with other people too. Self-awareness is an important part of mental, emotional, and spiritual health.

> Family: the people we laugh with, the people who sharpen us, the people who drive us crazy, the people we live out faith and homework and budgets with.

One Mother's Day I was leading worship at our church. I was getting baptized with my two precious kiddos at the end of the service (I know, it's too much, and my heart almost exploded). Since we attend a church plant, we typically borrow another church with a baptismal pool for baptism services. This was the first time we were holding the baptisms as part of the service.

As two of our pastors were getting the baptismal pool set up and filled, they were talking about the best way to handle the music, the baptisms, and the timing of everything. They were going around and around, having a hard time nailing things down. Something I have learned about myself over the years is that I'm the gal who will say, "If you're not going to make a choice, I will make it *for you*!"

So there I found myself, telling them what to do. Knowing my tendency, I quickly realized what I was doing. I acknowledged that I wasn't in charge of that situation and wouldn't even be singing during that time. I apologized and backed off. Ideally, I would have stopped myself before I butted in and forced my way on everyone . . . #goalz. But at least I was self-aware enough to hear that voice in my head saying, *You're doing it again . . .*

Personality tests are helpful in situations like this one, and they are even more beneficial in our closest and most intimate relationships.

Your flaws might not be immediately noticeable to an acquaintance or a friend, but since you spend the most time with your family, they see you at your best and your worst. It's so much easier to have grace and patience with someone when you understand their motivations and how they naturally navigate their world.

There are so many different personality tests you can explore to help you learn more about yourself and about the people you love.

You don't need to do all these personality tests at once—just pick one that resonates with you as a couple. Once you've taken the test, the most important part isn't about your specific results and how your personalities are similar or different; it's how you utilize and incorporate what you've learned. I think a huge aspect of our job as parents is to help our kids identify the gifts and traits they've been given by God. Using personality tests to help you

My Favorite Personality Tests

- **Enneagram:** This test explores not just behaviors but also core motivations, and it identifies nine different personality types. Find out more at the Enneagram Institute's site (enneagraminstitute.com).

- **Myers-Briggs Type Indicator:** This detailed personality test identifies sixteen different personality types, noting behaviors, strengths, and preferences. You can find out more at MBTI online (mbtionline.com).

- **DISC Assessment:** The DISC assessment measures interpersonal behavior and assigns each person a letter or combination of letters. You can find out more about this assessment at onlinedisctests.com.

- **Love Languages:** According to Gary Chapman, there are five primary ways people prefer to give and receive love. You can find out more in his book *The 5 Love Languages.*

- **Communication Styles:** A communication style is a unique way to listen, respond, make decisions, and solve problems. You can find out more at Straight Talk (communicationstyles.org).

understand those gifts will enable you to intentionally cultivate them in your children.

I've often heard that communication is the most important part of a relationship. There are two parts to communication: speaking and listening. When it comes to the way you talk to each other, the results of personality tests can help you communicate in a way that's most effective and meaningful for each of you.

If you've felt silenced or not listened to in your relationship, you can change that. It's never too late to communicate your needs. If this conversation feels too scary or confrontational to you, I recommend asking a pastor or counselor to help mediate.

Balancing Responsibilities

One of the biggest sources of conflict in marriage is the division of responsibilities. I want to say up front that there is no one right way to do this. So many factors go into assigning tasks, including work responsibilities, interests, skills, energy level, and time. What feels balanced for one couple might not work at all for another couple, and what works during one season may not be a fit during another life stage. What's important is that you can communicate about it honestly and that both parties feel like the workload is balanced. It's also important to note that this is not a once-and-done conversation; it's something you'll need to revisit as life changes. If things are unbalanced in this area, one person will eventually get burned out and will start to resent their spouse.

Chaz and I have been married for twelve years now, and we've settled into our roles in our home and our family, but it definitely took some time. Of the two of us, Chaz is the one who is clean and organized, and he cares about having a tidy space. (He joked the other night that he is the janitor of Olive You Whole because he cleans up behind me!) In addition to working around ten hours every day, he also works hard to keep our house clean. He picks up in the kitchen after dinner, puts dishes in the dishwasher and starts it, wipes the counters, and vacuums every night. He also manages our budget and finances (although nearly all our home bills are on autopay, so neither of us has to do that manually).

I, on the other hand, do the meal planning, grocery shopping, meal prepping, and cooking. I get the kids to school and take care of them and hang out with them when school isn't in session. I try to keep up with communication, work, and activities related to school and after-school activities. I buy the kids' clothes and shoes (though admittedly we don't get many!). I often do the laundry, though Chaz does too, and he usually helps me fold clothes and put them away.

> **Chores That Kids Can Do at Different Stages**
>
> - **Toddlers:** take dishes to the sink, help make their bed, pick up their toys, take off their shoes and put them away, put dirty clothes in the laundry basket
> - **Elementary school:** clean surfaces and mirrors, fill pets' food and water bowls, set the table, rinse their dishes and put them in the dishwasher
> - **Middle school/high school:** vacuum and sweep, do their laundry and put it away, clean toilets, clean showers and bathtubs, take out trash and recycling, empty the dishwasher

When your kids are in elementary school or older, they can help too! Our kiddos have chores every day and help us clean our home on the weekend. Now they know how to do their own laundry, fold it, and put it away.

If you're feeling like there's an imbalance in your family's responsibilities, have a conversation about it—first with your spouse and then with your children. Our friend told us about "Fair Play Deck" cards. They include all sorts of household chores and general life tasks, and you and your husband take the cards you usually have responsibility for. The goal isn't necessarily to have even stacks of cards since each one requires a different amount of time or effort, but it's a good way to get the conversation started. It's also eye opening because a lot of household activities have unspoken ownership. These cards allow you to claim different tasks and find a balance of assignments that works for both of you.

Finding Relational Rhythms

There's an interesting phenomenon about marriage: one minute you're newlyweds, and then you blink and you're twelve years in (I may or may not know from experience!). If you're not intentional, the time just flies by. Without guardrails and periodic check-ins, you will slowly grow apart instead of moving together in the same direction. As with an angle, even one degree of difference can result in a great distance after a long time.

Chaz and I realized that we needed to set up some intentional relational rhythms to keep our marriage on course. We've found it helpful to have daily, weekly, quarterly, and yearly checkpoints toward this goal.

Daily Check-Ins

This might sound obvious, but it's harder than it seems: you need to speak to your spouse every day. And this isn't just about who's picking up the kids or who's making dinner; it's about having real conversations. The reality is, between work, household duties, commitments, and kids' activities, it's easy to become ships passing in the night.

Connection is everything in marriage. When you settle for being busy during the week and waiting until the weekend to have meaningful conversations with your spouse, you're only connecting two-sevenths of the time. Out of 365 days in a year, that's a measly 104 days. We want something more than that, right?

If this sounds like a pipe dream, let me give you some tips to get started. I recommend setting a timer for five minutes each day—maybe when kids are at school or before they wake up or after they go to bed. Start with a simple question, like "What's going on in your life?" This doesn't need to be a formal, sit-down-at-the-table kind of situation. You can do this while on a walk, playing golf, or before you go to sleep. Remember, this connection time is not about household responsibilities, kids' activities, or logistics. This time is dedicated to what's going on in your thoughts and hearts, how you're truly doing, and how you can love each other well. I think after doing this for a while, you're going to start enjoying it and find that you want to keep going well past the five minutes!

Weekly Date Nights

Weekly date nights are like daily check-ins . . . but more fun! Getting out of the house provides fewer distractions and more opportunities for connection, so I recommend doing this every week if you can. I know going out can be expensive, so keep in mind this doesn't have to be a top-rated Michelin restaurant. Chaz is a pretty big stickler when it comes to the budget, so there are times when the date-night budget is low. For these times, we have a list of free and low-cost date options in our area. You might take a picnic to the park, go on a bike ride together, go on a hike, or just get coffee or dessert.

If you have littles, find a young babysitter who is eager for work! Or, to maximize your dating budget, do a swap with friends who have similar-aged kids. (Okay, I know this can be hard to find, but keep looking! It's worth the effort—who doesn't want free date nights?) We did this when we first moved to Denver—Chaz and I had two date nights a month, and our friends had two. We both loved the free babysitting, and it kept us committed to our date nights.

Quarterly Focus

Our friend Blake Howard runs a branding graphic design firm in Atlanta called Matchstic. Getting to the core of who you are and why you do what you do is at the heart of the corporate branding process. Blake took the discovery process he used with his clients and created a discovery process for individuals and couples. You figure out who you are, why you do what you do, and create your personal focus.

Having a clear quarterly focus has been incredibly helpful for me and Chaz. We knew a year before we moved from Atlanta to Denver that Chaz had gotten the fellowship and we'd be moving. About six months before moving, we had our quarterly focus discussion. There were so many costs associated with moving—not just the moving vans and the increased cost of living in Denver, but we also knew we wanted to get ski gear and ski passes. (Sheesh! Skiing is so expensive.)

Looking ahead, we knew this would be a season when we would need to prioritize making money. Chaz was in residency, so he had an opportunity to pick up extra shifts at the hospital. We agreed that for this three-month period, he would take on as many of these moonlighting shifts as he could.

It all comes down to having a clear purpose for the season and being in agreement with your spouse about that purpose. This decision to pick up extra shifts could have been beneficial or harmful for our family, depending on what we were trying to accomplish during that period. If our goal for that quarterly focus had been family time and Chaz picked up a bunch of extra shifts, that would have been super frustrating for me. But since this was what we'd agreed on for a specific length of time, I wasn't bitter, knowing he was doing what we'd agreed would benefit our family.

The next quarter fell during our last three months in Atlanta. Our focus was people (and food!). We wanted to spend as much time as possible with our community and family before heading out west. We also wanted to eat all the deliciousness Atlanta has to offer and visit the restaurants that had been on our "we really need to try that place sometime" list. It wasn't now or never, because we planned to return to Atlanta frequently. But now would definitely be easier than later, so why not now?

Having an agreed-upon focus helps us manage our priorities and our actions, and it helps us feel more aligned as a couple. If we had been blowing through cash eating out during our "make and save money" quarter, it would have been out of alignment with our goals. But given our goal for this quarter, it made sense for what we were trying to accomplish.

You can find a wellness-based quarterly focus guide inspired by Blake (with his permission) at oliveyouwhole.com/quarterly-focus. (Note that the first time you go through the process, it will take the longest, because you're filling out the "What are my two most important values?" and

"How are you uniquely positioned?" sections. These are similar to a DNA test—no need to redo them! When you come back to this practice each quarter, you just need to fill out the quarterly focus section.)

Year in Review

I believe an annual review is the most important practice a couple can have. This might look different for each couple, but here's what it looks like for Chaz and me. We usually take a trip for our anniversary, and we've found that's a great time for us to do our annual review. It usually takes us a few hours, so we'll go through the whole process in a morning. I recommend doing this when you can give it your undivided attention, so try to set aside time for just you and your spouse. This allows you to work through parts of your relationship, schedule, or habits that could be improved. You can do this year-in-review anytime.

I recommend keeping a list of action items to get you from where you are to where you want to be. I love this because it aligns closely with what I do as a health coach: bridge the gap between where we are and where we want to be.

This is your opportunity as a couple to get clear on this question: "Are we doing the things that are important to us?" We often assume something is a priority, but when we assess what we're actually doing, we realize we're not dedicating much of our time to it. This can be a brutal realization, but acknowledging the problem is the first step toward change.

When Chaz and I did our year in review recently, I realized that I wasn't exercising as much as I wanted to. So I asked myself some questions:

- Is this actually important to me, or do I just think it should be?
- If it's important to me, what is getting in the way of making this happen?
- How can I make this task or habit easier for myself?

I love our year in review because it feels like a fresh start. There are so many things Chaz and I want to improve about ourselves and our relationship, and this gives us a chance to reflect and find things we want to start doing, both individually and together.

You can find a printable version of our Relational Year in Review at oliveyouwhole.com/year-in-review. We generally spend about three hours filling out our evaluations and then talking about our results. If this sounds too intense, you can split it up into several different sections—whatever works for you and your spouse. We take some time to celebrate the things that are going well and then spend more time focusing on the areas we rated with room for improvement, whether we both ranked it low or just one of us did.

Once we've identified areas we'd like to work on, we make them actionable. We talk through why something might not be working. Are there barriers getting in the way? What small, actionable steps could we take to make this area better? We try to make the solutions as bite-sized as possible, and we commit to the smallest change that could have the biggest impact!

Creating a Culture of Honesty and Peace

Very early in our dating relationship, Chaz and I got into one of our first fights. I wish I could remember now what it was about, because I'm sure it was completely inconsequential. What I do remember is that Chaz did something that made me really mad on a Friday. I spent all weekend in a huff, trying to punish him by withholding myself from him. By the time Sunday rolled around, he finally was like, "WHAT IN THE WORLD, CAROLINE?!"

Now, I'm not one who loves to admit when I'm wrong, but this *one* time, I was. We talked through it, and I realized I had misunderstood the entire situation. So I'd emotionally punished Chaz for three days, but you know who else I punished with a not fun weekend? Myself!

Chaz suggested that from then on, we would adopt a twenty-four-hour rule. We decided we'd have twenty-four hours to bring up something the other person did or we could never bring it up again. Clearly, this was an exaggeration since there are times you need to bring up something from the past, but it helped us to set a default of not holding a grudge. Ephesians 4:26-27 says, "Do not let the sun go down on your anger, and give no opportunity to the devil" (ESV). We've found that it's better for us to bring up anything that happened the same day. This isn't meant to be a legalistic rule, just a goal to strive toward.

In our relationship, this has led to a culture of peace. It's a relief to know that Chaz isn't stewing on something I did. I trust that if I did something that offended him, he will tell me right away. When you regularly bring up small things in a relationship, it doesn't become a massive blowup fueled by years of bitter resentment. When you have a culture of immediate honesty, it builds a foundation of trust for the entire relationship.

Setting Parenting Goals

According to a Pew Research poll, 73 percent of Americans said one of their highest priorities is "spending time with family." In comparison, 32 percent said "practicing your religious faith" was important to them, and 31 percent valued "being physically active."[1] This prioritization of family shouldn't come as a surprise, because the benefits of a strong family unit are nearly endless.

But what does it mean to have a strong family? According to the website Raising Children, strong families provide warmth, care, positive attention, good communication, a predictable environment, and connections to other people outside the family.[2] Having healthy family connections gives children the confidence to try new things, knowing they have the support of those around them.

The first step of being intentional with your family involves thinking about your goals. It's impossible to prioritize everything, so you'll need to decide what's most important for your family's culture. For Chaz and me, our biggest goal for our kiddos (and ourselves) is that we love God and love other people. In order for that to be the case,

Chaz and I have to prioritize our relationship with God and model that for our kids. This is why we're committed to finding a church we adore (it took a while, but it was worth the effort!), and we go as often as we can. The kiddos love the community they have there, and we've surrounded ourselves with other people who love God and others too. At home, we try to pray with our kiddos, either at dinner or during bedtime snuggles. They get memory verses at church that we'll work on together (Chaz and I are excited that they're memorizing Scripture, and they're excited that when they get it right they get M&M's as a prize!).

One of our other goals in parenting is to raise kiddos who will become confident and capable adults. To me, that means helping them identify and embrace their God-given gifts and develop their strengths. We're constantly trying to point out the positive attributes we see in them. It's as simple as saying, "Wow, Owen. That was super generous of you to offer our guests one of your stuffies. You are a generous little boy!" I truly believe self-confidence starts in the home. We have the opportunity to build our children up instead of dragging them down.

Chaz and I believe a huge part of parenting is teaching our children the skills of adulting, as annoying as those responsibilities can be! We want our kids to learn how to work hard, anticipate and avoid problems, and solve problems when they arise. They earn money by doing chores like cleaning and laundry, learn how to use their money wisely, and practice important relationship skills like forgiveness and reconciliation. If we don't teach our children how to be responsible while they're in our home, how will they know how to do these things when they're out on their own?

I recommend sitting down with your spouse and choosing your goal or goals for raising your children. These goals should be in line with your overall family values. You might want your children to be kind to everyone they encounter. Or you might want your kids to participate in athletics. One of the keys is to be sure you and your spouse are in agreement about your goals for your family and your children.

Creating a Family Mission Statement

Once you've nailed down your goals for your parenting and for your family, it's time to write a family mission statement. This statement outlines your core values and what your family is on this planet to accomplish. To create your family's mission statement, start with the values you nailed down in chapter 6, combined with the parenting goals you decided on, and create a rough draft. This may be something you revise as your children get older and as you refine your values, but remember—done is better than perfect.

It's best if the entire family participates in crafting your mission statement. It should be collaborative, not dictated, if you want buy-in from everyone. You can dedicate an evening to this event, and make it fun! (Homemade pizza night? Camping in the backyard? Get creative—just make sure it fits your family!) Explain in detail what a family mission statement is so everyone understands the objective. Make sure everyone knows that their input is important. This will help them feel heard and like a critical part of your family unit.

As you brainstorm, make a list of suggestions, then work together to finalize the list to the top three or four most important points. While it's fun to get your family mission statement printed out or framed, keep in mind that it's not set in stone. It can grow and change as your family does.

Your family mission statement leans heavily on your family values. Some families choose to include individual goals and action items like "We adventure often!" or "We strive to be brave and courageous!" There is no right way—your family mission statement will be unique to your family.

Here's our family mission statement: "We exist to be loving, kind, and encouraging—within our family and to everyone we interact with." When one of our kids (or one of us—let's be honest) isn't very encouraging, we say, "What's our family mission statement?" They repeat it. Then we will say, "Was the way you just talked to that person very encouraging?" They say no, and then (usually on their own), they'll apologize.

Once you've all memorized your family mission statement, you can remind each other when someone acts outside of it.

Spending Intentional Time Together

If the statistics are right, we all want to spend time together as family. Unfortunately, it's not always that easy—it's something we have to fight for. We get bogged down by busyness and activities, and before we know it, we hardly see the other people in our family, especially as our kids get older! It takes intentionality to prioritize family time as your children grow, but I'm here to tell you: it *is* possible!

Our family uses a few different strategies to make sure we spend time together. We set aside daily and weekly times to be together, along with bigger chunks of time each year. You may find other rhythms that work well for your family, but this will give you a place to begin.

Family Dinners

When I was a child, my dad's biggest priority was for us to eat dinner together. He'd heard studies about what makes adults successful, and eating dinner as a family was the number one factor for success later in life. It turns out, he was right.

When you eat together as a family, your kiddos establish better nutrition habits that have lasting effects.[3] It has also been shown that eating meals together as a family reduces the chance of weight gain and obesity ten years later. Talk about giving your kids something that will last![4]

Regular family dinners also have academic, social, and emotional benefits. In the book *The Power of Habit*, Charles Duhigg says, "Studies have documented that families who habitually eat dinner together seem to raise children with better homework skills, higher grades, greater emotional control, and more confidence."[5] Family dinners are associated with lower rates of depression, anxiety, eating disorders, substance abuse, tobacco use, and early teenage pregnancy, as well as higher rates of resilience and higher self-esteem.[6] But even with all these benefits, according to the Family Dinner Project, only 30 percent of families eat together regularly.[7]

Okay, so maybe you're convinced that family meals are a priority. But what do you talk about when you all sit down at the table?

I want to provide you with a tried-and-true strategy for making dinnertime conversation easy and more meaningful! If you're tired of the "'How was your day?' 'Good'" routine, this "rose/bud/thorn" game is worth a try. Our beloved small group in Atlanta introduced us to this idea (and I still play it with them via group text thread!).

Here's how it works: each person shares their rose, bud, and thorn for the day. Your rose is the best thing that happened to you that day, your bud is something you're looking forward to, and your thorn is something bad that happened to you. On my own, I probably wouldn't think to ask, "Did anything terrible happen to you today?" But having that "thorn" conversation has given Chaz and me insight into our kiddos' struggles over the years. Without this prompting, I think we would have missed a lot of these moments.

This game provides an opportunity to connect with your kiddos and make sure they know you care about who they are and that you value what's important to them.

Kid Dates

We do individual dates with the kids, and we've been amazed at the way it fills up their little cups. We only have two kiddos, so Chaz and I will each take a kid at the same time. If we have limited time, we take them to the same breakfast place and sit at different tables. You can also let each kid decide something fun they want to do (this can be something free, or you can give them a budget!). If you have more than two kids, keep a schedule of whose turn it is to have a mommy date or daddy date. There's no one way to do this—the important thing is that each child has one-on-one time with each parent.

Kids feel so special when they get individual attention like this.

We let the kids decide where we eat or what we do. During this time, we often find out new details about their lives that we haven't heard before, good and bad. While it's important to spend time together as a family, it's also vital to connect with kids one-on-one and have fun with them!

Family Trips

I love traveling as a family for many reasons. For one thing, it gets us out of our little neighborhood and exposes us to other cultures, different parts of history, and new environments. We especially enjoy visiting national parks. These trips have opened our eyes to the fact that there are grasslands, forests, deserts, caves, raging rivers, mountain ranges, and Everglades all within our own country. We want our kids to know that not everyone looks like them or has the same culture, religion, or way of doing things, and that everyone is made by God and precious in his sight.

Another reason we enjoy traveling is because it takes us out of our comfort zone and routines. When we travel, we bring along games and have game nights. We spend quality time together, making memories.

I want to note here that travel doesn't have to be a grand international adventure. It can take a lot of forms and is possible even without spending a lot of time and money. As you begin planning a trip, set a budget and think about how much time you want to be gone. Consider how your kiddos do with traveling, set a number of hours you'll travel, and then see where you could go within that radius. To keep it budget friendly, you can go grocery shopping before you leave and pack meals and snacks for the road, or buy food when you arrive so you don't have to eat out for every meal. We often stay at extended-stay hotels because they have a kitchenette and we can make our meals "in," which ends up being both healthier and more affordable. You can also stay with friends or family to save on hotel costs.

Regardless of where you go, what you do, or how much you spend,

I think you'll find that traveling together is worth it, and the memories are priceless.

Creating a Safe Haven

Our kiddos learn a lot of their emotional intelligence from us, their parents. No pressure, right? But that doesn't mean we need to be perfect. They gain emotional skills when they see us getting it right—and also when we get it wrong and then model how to apologize and repair the relationship.

One of our big priorities as a family is to practice asking for forgiveness. Chaz and I are *not* perfect parents. I have the patience of a flea . . . so if I snap at our kids or yell at them, I try to go back and apologize to them once I'm calm. Owning our mistakes and asking for forgiveness is so important, because our kids are watching and learning from us, even when we don't realize it. It might be tempting to try to maintain a steely "parents are always right" disposition, but that will be harmful to your children—and your relationship—in both the short term and the long term.

> ### When to Get Professional Help
>
> I want to note here that there is a time and place to end a relationship. If you don't feel safe in your relationship, it's time to seek professional help. No one should make you feel belittled. No one should touch you in a way you don't consent to, especially if they're harming you or forcing you to do something you don't want to. If you or someone you know may be experiencing abuse, please reach out to the National Domestic Violence Hotline at 800-799-7233. They are open 24-7 and can accommodate more than two hundred languages. This is a safe, nonjudgmental place to share your story and get the resources you need. It is never too late to get help and to get out if you need to.

It can be hard to navigate our own feelings and our children's feelings at times, especially since we're often feeling big feelings at the same time! In previous generations, many parents instructed their children not to feel what were deemed "negative" feelings: "Don't be sad!" "Don't cry!" "Come on, get over it already!" Instead of labeling feelings as bad,

k

or punishing or discouraging children from experiencing these emotions, it's important to teach our children how to feel their feelings and provide a safe space for them to do so.

Dr. Becky Kennedy, a clinical psychologist and the founder of Good Inside, encourages this as a value in our homes: "All feelings are allowed, even the ones we don't expect." This concept not only helps children regulate their emotions but will continue to help them regulate their emotions as adults. Dr. Becky adds, "We can only learn to regulate the feelings we allow ourselves to have."[8]

Dr. Jill Bolte Taylor describes how fleeting emotions are in her book *My Stroke of Insight*. Once an emotion such as anger is triggered in the brain, chemicals are released throughout the body. Within ninety seconds, the chemical component has completely dissipated from the blood, and if we remain angry after that, it's a matter of choice. This information is helpful as we process emotions: "The healthiest way I know how to move through an emotion effectively is to surrender completely to that emotion when its loop of physiology comes over me. I simply resign to the loop and let it run its course for ninety seconds. Just like children, emotions heal when they are heard and validated. Over time, the intensity and frequency of these circuits usually abate."[9]

I use the ninety-second rule to my benefit: I simply breathe through an emotion for ninety seconds and see how I'm feeling when that time is up. Of course, there are times when we've been wounded deeply and we need to navigate these situations with a more in-depth conversation, listening, and asking for forgiveness.

Family Challenge

Beginner challenge: Take a chunk of time and dedicate it to writing your family mission statement! Remember to let everyone in the family chime in—it's only complete when everyone loves it! Once it's complete, consider printing it out, framing it, and putting it somewhere special.

Intermediate challenge: Set up a date with each of your kiddos. You could take them out for a date, a meal, or a fun activity. For a budget-friendly option, you could even do a fun activity together at home like play board games or do a craft.

Advanced challenge: Set up a babysitter for a weekly date night. You might consider a babysitter swap with another family—take turns going on a date and babysitting. Make a list of restaurants you'd like to go to and activities you'd like to do together so you'll have ideas when date night rolls around.

PART FOUR

Faith

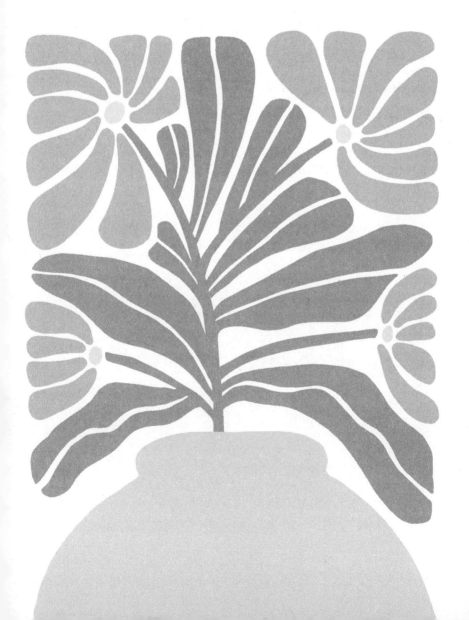

CHAPTER 11

SABBATH

The Sabbath is only a day, yet it is the gateway to another eon that cannot be entered by any other door.

DAN ALLENDER

I like to say I have loved Jesus from the womb. My family went to church every Sunday morning and Wednesday night since before I was born. Yet somehow in all that churchgoing, I heard about the Sabbath only a few times in passing. It was described as a day of mandated rest for the Israelites that had nothing to do with our lives now. It seemed to fall into the same category as the thousands of laws in Leviticus that had been fulfilled by Christ. In other words, we were no longer bound by this commandment.

But let's take a step back and get some background on this topic. The Hebrew word *Shabbat* literally means "to stop" or "to rest." Its roots go all the way back to the first story in the Bible. "By the seventh day God had finished the work he had been doing; so on the seventh day he rested from all his work. Then God blessed the seventh day and made it holy, because on it he rested from all the work of creating that he had done" (Genesis 2:2-3).

After creating the world, God stopped. He rested and delighted in and with his creation. An article at BibleProject.com points out the connection between God resting himself and then settling his people. After God rested on the seventh day, he created humans and then immediately "rests them" or "settles them" in the Garden with him (see Genesis 2:15). "God leads by example as he rests from work (*shabbat*), and then he dwells (*nuakh*) with his people."[1] Now that Jesus has entered our world as God incarnate, he is the way we receive the invitation to fully rest in him.

In case all this Bible talk feels like a lot for you, let me stop for a moment and say this: the Sabbath is for *everyone*. Regardless of your faith or lack thereof, the invitation to the Sabbath as a way of life is extended to you too. We were all made to rest—heart, mind, body, and soul.

And if you grew up in an environment where the Sabbath was motivated by legalism instead of freedom, I want to assure you that God's heart in this is not to create more obligations to follow. Here's Jesus' heart: "Come to me, all you who are weary and burdened, and I will give you rest. Take my yoke upon you and learn from me, for I am gentle and humble in heart, and you will find rest for your souls" (Matthew 11:28-29). These words are recorded right before Jesus was confronted about the way he observed the Sabbath. The people had become burdened by the thousands of laws and requirements about the Sabbath added by the religious leaders, who had missed the heart of it! Jesus offers himself as the solution: he is the Sabbath rest God promised to us.

What Is the Sabbath?

The Sabbath consists of three elements: stop working, dwell with God, and take delight!

The Sabbath is more than just a weekend or a day off. Without the intention and structure of a Sabbath, a day during the weekend can be packed to the brim with brunch, practices and activities, football games, grocery shopping, and cleaning, all while keeping up with our phones and email. Sometimes a weekend can be even more exhausting than a weekday!

Eugene Peterson, a pastor and the author of *The Message*, says that a day off is a "bastard Sabbath."[2] Without a deeper purpose to our Sabbath, we miss out on its true intention. The truth is, the things we assume will recharge us often are the very things that make us feel grouchy and unsatisfied—and even more drained than before.

So many of us are exhausted beyond measure. We are overbooked, overworked, and over-committed. That's a recipe for burnout—which is exactly where many of us find ourselves! Sometimes it seems like there's no solution to the madness. But I think there is. The answer is not a new fad or a life hack or a quick fix. It's an ancient practice called the Sabbath.

> The Sabbath consists of three elements: stop working, dwell with God, and take delight!

When God declared the Sabbath day, he commanded us to cease all work, rest with him, and delight in him and his creation (see Exodus 20:8-11). This may look different for each person and each family, but the heart behind it is the same: it gives us the chance to rest, refresh, and recharge.

A few years ago, Chaz listened to an interview with John Mark Comer about his book *The Ruthless Elimination of Hurry* on the podcast *Dad Tired*. My husband said to me, "Babe, I think I'm going to read this book. Comer practices a Sabbath where he doesn't work at all for twenty-four hours, he fully stops at stop signs, and he doesn't get into the shortest line at the grocery store. Want to read it with me?"

There I was, with two small kiddos, trying to fit *all* the things into my day—running a business, writing a cookbook, washing dishes, doing laundry—and this man was standing in front of me suggesting that I learn how to slow down? How could I slow down? Even the idea of reading the book was off-putting to me. I didn't want to slow down—I didn't have time to slow down!

So Chaz listened to the book on his own and absolutely inhaled it.

He came back to me a second time and said, "Caroline, I felt like I was trying to lead our family spiritually by suggesting that we read this book together, and you shot me down."

I was speechless, because I hadn't realized that was what I was doing. And now I felt like a total jerk! So I said, "Okay, next time, if that's what you're doing, can you *lead* with that, and I'll say yes? Yes, I will read this book with you."

So Chaz read the book again, with me this time, and it changed our lives. The world had pushed its "hustle and hurry" narrative on me, and I had bought it completely, hook, line, and sinker. Comer showed us the easy yoke of Jesus that had been available to us the whole time. I realized my hesitation came because I had a misguided understanding of what the Sabbath was. I only understood the *stop* part of it: stop working, stop spending, stop moving fast. I didn't realize that the Sabbath is truly an invitation into sheer delight.

You know your breaking point? That point where all semblance of patience is gone, and you forget you don't yell, because you are yelling now? Let's call that 100. When you're living a busy, overstretched life, you may wake up every single day at an 80. You get negative feedback from your boss, a kid forgets their lunch box, and your dinner plans fall through so now you have to make dinner. It's been a *day*. It doesn't take much to push you to 100. (If you can't tell, I'm speaking from personal experience here.) What Sabbath does for me is bring my starting point down to 0.

For our family, Sabbath is a day to reconnect. We connect with God, we connect with one another, and we connect as a couple. While it seems like what we do and don't do on Sabbath changes from week to week, this might give you an idea of what this looks like for us. We say yes to worship, prayer, solitude, rest, naps, delicious food, family games, time in nature, community with our dearest friends, and sweet treats to remember the goodness of God. We say no to work (and even thinking or talking about work), housework, our personal to-do lists, screens, buying things, as much cooking as possible, and anything that feels burdensome. Without all these distractions and with the emphasis of rest, we like to say that Sabbath feels like two whole days. Somehow the day goes on and on, but in the best way. We're doing all our favorite things, and our souls come alive again. After a twenty-four-hour Sabbath, it feels like my barrel of patience has been filled up again. I'm reminded of the things that are most important to me and the values we hold dear.

Time is the only thing in life we can't get back. Even the richest people in the world can't buy time. But on the Sabbath, time slows down. And in a way, you *can* get time back. Scientists believe that one of the factors that contributes to people in the Loma Linda, California, "blue zone" living longer (9.5 years for men and 6.1 years for women) is keeping the Sabbath.[3] Our bodies and minds simply weren't made to operate nonstop—we need to reset regularly if we want them to run optimally.

What If I'm Too Busy to Take a Sabbath?

You might hear the word Sabbath and think, *But I can't because . . .* You may have one million reasons for not practicing the Sabbath. The most common is "But I'm so busy!" That may be true, but that's actually the point!

According to a recent Gallup survey, the average full-time employee works forty-four hours per week, and 41 percent of employees work more than forty-five hours per week.[4] The International Labour Organization found that the yearly hours worked in the US is greater than the other countries they surveyed, including Australia, the UK, Sweden, Belgium, France, and Germany.[5] More than half of Americans report having PTO they haven't used, and 27.2 percent of paid time off goes completely unused every year.[6] Part of the problem is that busyness, productivity, and overworking are celebrated in our culture. After living for so long on an adrenaline high of working constantly, it can feel countercultural and unnatural to devote an entire day to produce *nothing*.

If you don't think you have time for the Sabbath, let me present a revolutionary idea to you: God rested.

Whatever your *But I . . .* response is to the Sabbath, my response is, "But God."

Y'all, the creator of the universe stopped everything he was doing to rest. And let's be clear here: it wasn't because creating the world made him tired. No, he saw that what he made was good, and he took one-seventh of his time to delight in his creation.

Then he commanded us to do the same.

We rest and delight for an entire day, producing absolutely nothing, trusting that God will provide. The Sabbath strengthens our ability to trust God not just on the Sabbath but on the other six days of the week too. He always has provided—and he always will.

Truly, the Sabbath is an act of humility that takes us out of the center of our universe and puts God there instead.

> The Sabbath is an act of humility that takes us out of the center of our universe and puts God there instead.

How Do You Prepare for the Sabbath?

Our family celebrates a Sabbath during the traditional time frame of Friday evening to Saturday evening. Some people choose to mark the Sabbath on Sunday, when they go to church and worship God. Since Chaz and I frequently volunteer at church, Sundays can feel like work to us, so we rest the day before instead.

If part of your goal for the Sabbath is to have a day without work, household chores, or technology, you'll need to plan ahead a bit. I've found that the more preparations I do the day before our Sabbath, the sweeter the rest and enjoyment of the Sabbath is.

We typically clean the house before our Sabbath, because it's more relaxing to rest in a clean environment. This doesn't have to be the world's deepest clean, but I try to check the laundry to see if anything needs to be done (for example, clothes for sports games or church). We also try to tidy up the main shared spaces. We empty the dishwasher so we can put dishes in the dishwasher instead of letting them pile up in the sink.

You'll need to consider what you'll eat on the Sabbath and prepare ahead of time. We typically make stew during the day on Friday, and then keep it in the Instant Pot bowl in the fridge until right before the Sabbath starts. Then I put the bowl in the Instant Pot, set it on slow cook for fourteen hours on a two-hour delay (it stays cold enough before it cooks). That timing works perfectly so we can eat it for lunch on our Sabbath. And I tell you what—the meat is fall-apart tender and delicious!

If you choose not to use your phone during the Sabbath, you will need to communicate plans with anyone outside your family in advance. If you want to invite someone to join your Sabbath meal, do so beforehand and let them know about what time you'll be turning off your phone. The same goes for any plans on the Sabbath day.

Just as the Sabbath will look different for each person and family, everyone's preparations will vary too. Just try to look ahead to your Sabbath day and think about what might need to be done in advance so you can relish your rest.

How Do You Practice the Sabbath?

Scripture emphasizes over and over that the Sabbath is more about the heart and intent rather than making thousands of legalistic rules. But here are some guidelines that our family follows for our Sabbath.

Stop Working

Generally, we don't do any work, and we try not to even think about work (which is hard, I know!). We also avoid doing house chores, so we try to do our weekly cleaning the day before the Sabbath. We don't really have a yard, but we also don't do yard work or gardening, and I water my plants before the Sabbath begins. We also try to cook before the Sabbath. We avoid spending money on the Sabbath, and we try to stay away from anything that would make us want more things (like magazines). We are off technology as much as possible, though typically one of us will keep a phone on us in case of an emergency.

A note on technology. Many of us are inextricably tied to our phones—it's as if our phones are extra appendages. We feel like we've lost a limb when our phone is off or out of reach. If the thought of giving up your phone for a day makes you break out in hives or start hyperventilating a bit, that's probably evidence that taking a day off from technology would be good for you. We often think that our phones are providing something beneficial for us, and of course, phones aren't all bad. But it's eye opening to discover how we fill our time when we're not picking up our phone every spare moment and how much more fulfilling our day can be without it.

We recently took our kids on a "last hurrah" summer trip to a hotel with a water park near our house. I was shocked by how many water-proof phone cases I saw. Instead of relaxing on the lazy river, teenagers were filming content underwater. I couldn't help but wonder if these kids were missing out on the joy of the moment in favor of creating their next TikTok video.

We all need breaks from technology. This requires intentionality, because our phones are literally created to make us addicted. In addition to having a no-phone-zone on our Sabbath, we also try to make our smartphones as dumb as possible. Chaz and I have removed nearly all notifications—we try to get pinged and dinged as seldom as possible. We may be a little more

Things You Might Say No to on the Sabbath

- Work
- Chores and housework
- Yard work/gardening
- Cooking
- Spending money
- Technology

Things You Might Say Yes to on the Sabbath

- Journal
- Pray
- Practice silence and solitude
- Listen to worship music
- Feast and eat sweet treats
- Rest
- Nap
- Make love with your spouse
- Go on a walk or a hike
- Get out in nature
- Do something creative
- Spend time with your favorite people
- Play games

out of touch and a little less reachable this way, but it's worth it for our sanity.

Dwell with God

I used to assume that spending time with God meant only two things: reading the Bible and praying. It wasn't until we began John Mark Comer's study *Practicing the Way* that I learned about other forms of spiritual formation practices: silence, solitude, dealing with your past, fasting, forgiveness, community, and more.

My pastor, Megan Hermes (who also happens to be one of my best friends), refers to these ways of spending time with God as a menu. There are many ways to grow closer to God. But you don't need to feel pressure to do all of them on a given Sabbath; just pick one or two that resonate with you and your season of life. We all grow closer to God in different ways, and we need different practices at different times.

Are you in an intense season of work or caregiving? Don't add to your stress by viewing the Sabbath as one more thing on your to-do list. If you can't dedicate an entire day to Sabbath, do your best! Maybe it simply looks like listening to worship music throughout the day. The Sabbath should be peaceful and restful, so see how you can make these principles work in your current season of life.

Regardless of the avenue you choose, one of the main goals of the Sabbath is to dwell with God. Something to note here is that it's often the things that seem completely contrary to our personality that are often the most beneficial for us. It will probably be a lifelong battle for me to hold my tongue. For that reason, silence and solitude are two practices that have been incredibly life changing for me. Don't be scared to try new things—you might be surprised by how much you enjoy them!

Delight in God

As an Enneagram 7, I am all for fun, joy, and excitement, so I love that delight is our job on the Sabbath! One of the reasons I was hesitant to practice the Sabbath at first was because it seemed like it would be a dull, boring day. While spiritual formation practices are an important part of the day, the Sabbath isn't just about sitting silently in prayer, meditation, and fasting. No, it's a day of delight! Whatever it is you love doing, that's what you should prioritize on your Sabbath.

Isaiah 58:13-14 says, "If you keep your feet from breaking the Sabbath and from doing as you please on my holy day, *if you call the Sabbath a delight* and the LORD's holy day honorable, and if you honor it by not going your own way and not doing as you please or speaking idle words, then you will find your joy in the LORD" (emphasis added). Delight means doing the things that bring you most joy. And that will be different for each of us! For our family, that includes things like inviting our friends over for a Sabbath feast, going on hikes and seeing God in the beautiful Colorado mountains, and playing outside with our kids. Whatever brings us joy, we try to prioritize!

Delight goes beyond doing things you enjoy. We also celebrate with what we eat and drink. Chaz and I don't typically drink much, but after studying the history of the Sabbath, we've decided to drink a glass of wine on the Sabbath as a way to mark the celebration. It's also customary to eat a sweet treat as a reminder of the sweetness of God. Our favorite sweet treat for Sabbath is to put cookie dough in a skillet, then bake it in the oven. We cook it until it's *almost* done but still gooey in the middle, and then we serve it with ice cream.

What If Taking a Sabbath Feels Hard?

When you start practicing a Sabbath, don't be surprised if negative emotions arise. It is deeply ingrained in our culture to hustle, and it can feel like a crisis of identity when we're not producing. Who are we if we're not contributing or checking something off a list?

This is one of the reasons the Sabbath is so helpful—it reorients us to who we are at the core, not what we do. When we practice the Sabbath, it might involve taking away some of our typical coping mechanisms, such as checking our phone, shopping, or working. It's healthy to learn to deal with our emotions head-on when they come up. It may force us to learn new, healthier rhythms instead.

Part of practicing the Sabbath also involves setting boundaries. For one thing, you'll need to set a firm boundary with yourself to keep your phone off that day. Then you'll have to explain to your friend why you weren't able to text back right away. It might mean not going to an event on your day of rest and then explaining that to the host. If you're not used to setting and keeping boundaries, this can involve a learning curve.

It might get harder before it gets easier, but don't be alarmed—this is just part of the process! Take some time to journal about how you're feeling, and keep track of your progress. I promise, it will be worth it!

I've heard people argue that since Jesus came to fulfill the law, we don't "have to" keep the Sabbath. But I think that argument misses the point. Imagine if your kids went to school seven days a week and then you offered to take them to Disney World for the most magical day of their lives, and they said, "But do we have to?"

If our focus is on whether a Sabbath is required, we clearly have never experienced the *gift* that the Sabbath is.

I believe that God created a rhythm to the universe. Just as he created gravity with certain parameters ("What goes up must come down"), he created humans to survive at a certain pace ("Any human who goes without stopping will eventually run out of steam"). We weren't made for eighty-hour workweeks. We weren't made to work and think about work 24-7. We need an entire day to be reminded that our value is not in our work but in who we are.

> ## Ideas for Your Sabbath Meal
>
> One thing that helps the Sabbath become part of the fabric of your family is to create your own rituals and traditions that go with it. Here are some ideas, inspired by traditional Jewish Sabbath practices.
>
> - Say a blessing over your Sabbath meal (consider doing a call-and-response prayer, if you're feeling ambitious!).
> - Light candles at your meal (consider lighting one for each member of the family).
> - Say a blessing over your children at the end of your meal (consider reciting Numbers 6:24-26).
> - Make challah bread in advance and eat it at your meal (this is a Jewish Sabbath tradition).

So, do you have to take a Sabbath? Nope. Will something else stop you if you don't take the time to stop yourself? Yes, I think so.

The Sabbath isn't something you *have* to do; it's an invitation. You're invited into true rest. You're given a taste of heaven on earth. I think that once you acquire a taste for this kind of rest, you'll begin to crave it every week.

Sabbath Challenge

Beginner challenge: Set aside a few hours one day each week to not work at all—not for your job, your home, or your personal life. Take this time to stop, rest, worship, and delight. This is a little taste of the Sabbath, and once you try it, I know you'll want more!

Intermediate challenge: Set aside one day a week for a month and declare it a technology-free day. You may find it hard to "detox" at first, so I recommend making a list of things you enjoy that you can do instead of looking at your phone. This can be challenging, so I recommend turning it off and putting it in a drawer, out of sight!

Advanced challenge: Practice a full-fledged Sabbath day. Commit to not working one day a week for a month. This includes work you get paid for, as well as work around the house. Think of things you enjoy that you could do during that time instead. Try to find ways you feel close to God, and bring those things into your Sabbath.

CHAPTER 12

FINDING YOUR PURPOSE

*Living on purpose is the only way to really
live. Everything else is just existing.*

RICK WARREN

There's no greater joy than feeling passionate and purposeful about what
you do every day and what you're working toward. But how do you
figure out what that is? In this chapter, we'll talk about how to narrow
down your interests, skills, and passions to build the life you desire.

Scientists have found that feeling like you have a sense of purpose is
an indicator of healthy aging, promoting longevity and lowering your
mortality risk.[1] The thing about purpose is that it doesn't just happen
automatically. Either you choose your destination or you will end up
wherever life takes you. But no matter where you are on this journey
toward meaning or what obstacles and roadblocks you've faced along
the way, I truly believe you will do something with this beautiful life of
yours! You are on a moving pathway, like the ones at an airport, heading
toward a life of meaning.

The days are long, but the years are short. As a wellness coach, I've
had so many women come to me after their babies leave the nest and ask,

"Where did my life go?" As women, we have a tendency to get so involved in our kiddos' lives that we sometimes get lost and stop living our own.

Someone without a purpose is like a rubber duck that has been dropped off in the ocean. It might float along in the ocean for a while. It might even go to some really cool places. But without a sense of purpose, it's meandering at best.

One of the markers of someone without purpose is constant change. They're always looking for the next best thing to give them a sense of purpose. They might keep changing jobs, trying to find one that fits. They move on to a new significant other, hoping this one is finally "the one." They might change churches, move to different cities, pick up new hobbies, or find a new friend group. None of these things are bad on their own, but when there's a pattern of seeking external change to fill an inner void, it's often the result of an underlying lack of vision or purpose.

> Either you choose your destination or you will end up wherever life takes you.

What Is a Life Purpose?

We are created with a deep need for meaning in our lives, but this will look different for each person. There are certain callings God has given all of us: to love him, to love others, and to obey his commands. But I believe he also has plans that are unique to the way he has wired us as individuals. He instilled unique gifts in each of us, and he wants to use those gifts for his Kingdom. Ephesians 2:10 says, "We are God's handiwork, created in Christ Jesus to do good works, which God prepared in advance for us to do."

There are a lot of mountain trails here in Keystone, Colorado. People love to bike the Breck Keystone Loop—an eighteen-mile trail that goes from Keystone all the way to the famous ski town of Breckenridge. Imagine if you were dropped off by a helicopter onto Keystone Mountain with the sole objective of finding the Breck Keystone Loop trail. There's not just one path to get there—you could make your way to the trail via any number of routes. If someone told you there was only one right way to get there, you'd probably be sweating, right?

This is how people often approach your life's purpose—that there's just one right path for you to take. Either you're living it out or you're missing it entirely, aimlessly lost in the woods. I believe there isn't just one path we need to find and then stay on it our whole life. That sounds like a lot of unnecessary pressure!

If I didn't own Olive You Whole, helping people live their healthiest lives, who knows what path I might have followed? Maybe I would have been a singer, a travel agent, a flight attendant, a therapist, a pastor, an interior designer, or an event planner. (I recognize how very Enneagram 7 it is to have such a varied list!) I don't think any of these callings is more worthy than another. If I'd ended up as a wedding planner instead of a health coach and author, I believe God could have used my gifts in that capacity too. Who knows, I might even have a second career in one of these other fields one day!

Finding your purpose is not like playing a game of "Where's Waldo?," where you'll lose if you don't find that one elusive plan for your life. Instead, you can just try to find *a* purpose for your life—one that fits what you love and the way you're wired.

I also recognize that we don't always have the luxury of having a job that fits our passions. Sometimes we have to work simply to pay the bills and make ends meet. But even if we don't have our dream job, there are still ways we can use our unique giftings and passions to create meaning in our lives. While 70 percent of people find meaning in their jobs, this is a relatively recent privilege, and it's possible to find meaning outside your work as well.[2] According to Pew Research Center, people find meaning and fulfillment in these areas: spending time with family, being outdoors and experiencing nature, spending time with friends, practicing their religious faith, and doing volunteer work.[3] Maybe you work full time, but you find your biggest purpose in raising your family. Or maybe your volunteer work is what you're most passionate about. The key is to find what God is calling you to that makes you feel alive and then pursue it!

What If You Could Do Anything?

If you don't currently feel like you're living your purpose, you may still have an inkling about what you enjoy and what your passions are. If you could do anything with your one life, what would it be? Maybe there's something you've seen others doing and you thought, *Wow, that looks so rewarding. I would love to do that!*

Your purpose may be tied in with your job or what you have training or education in, but it can also just be something that fills you up. In college, I got degrees in graphic design and advertising, which I enjoy, but the thing that really drives me is a passion for health and wellness and food. This is something that has followed me for decades, and I haven't been able to shake it! Do you have a nagging sense that there's something you were made to do—that God has more for your life than you're experiencing right now? If so, it's time to explore that feeling and see if you can find your God-given purpose!

What Do You Love?

Recently, I was sharing with my friend Alissa that there is a sentence that rings in my heart and mind on repeat: *Help more people.* I was feeling discouraged, wondering if I was helping enough people. I felt like I was failing.

"How many collective followers do you have?" she asked.

"I don't know . . . around 100,000."

"How many people have been to your website?"

"Millions," I said.

"What about Pinterest? How many people have seen your pins?"

"Gosh, probably hundreds of millions?" I replied.

"I'm really glad God has given you this clear calling. I think it pushes you to keep going. But you know what? Not only do I not have that same calling, I've literally never had that thought! Not once."

Her insight helped me to gain some perspective. Not everyone in the world is supposed to reach a wide audience. That's my personal calling—one I've committed myself to. And I believe that if we get still and quiet enough, God will show each of us how he wants to use us and the unique gifts and passions he's instilled in us. I firmly believe these callings don't originate with us.

It's not just God. And it's not just us. Like all of Christianity, it's God plus us, working in harmony.

American author and theologian Frederick Buechner said, "The kind of work God usually calls you to is the kind of work (a) that you need most to do and (b) that the world most needs to have done. . . . The place God calls you to is the place where your deep gladness and the world's deep hunger meet."[4] Knowing that God is the one who puts the desires in our hearts in the first place, what brings you "deep gladness"? What do you love to do?

You may be in a season of your life when you have to work three jobs and have absolutely zero time to daydream. Or maybe you're a mom of young kids with spit-up splattered on your shirt and you have no space to consider what you want or would love to do right now. If that's where you're at, try to stick with me for a little bit!

If you had an entire day to do literally whatever you wanted, with no budget, no time restraints, and no child-care considerations, what would bring you the most joy?

Take some time to write down your answers, and try not to filter your response. Don't write what you think you should do or what your friends or family would say; just write what comes to you. If you're having trouble, here are some questions to prompt more ideas:

- When was the last time you laughed really hard?
- Think of a time you felt overwhelmingly happy. What prompted this feeling?
- How do you spend your money? What insight does this give you about the things you prioritize?
- When you have unexpected free time, what are you most excited to do?

Here are my answers: I love food. I enjoy trying new foods and making up new recipes. I am always thinking about health and wellness—new trends, supplements, longevity hacks, how to be healthy, and how I can share this information with others. I love creative things—crafting, painting, writing music, and playing the piano. I love talking to people and helping them find actionable answers to their problems, whether health-related or emotional. I love being active: swimming, riding my bike, rock climbing, hiking, running, and going on walks with friends. I love the beach—anything and everything about lying in the sand and playing in the ocean waves. I love traveling and exploring new places, new people, and new cultures.

When you're finished jotting down your list of things you enjoy, take some time to look it over and see if any threads jump out at you.

What Did You Enjoy as a Child?

Thinking back on your childhood can give you clues into your true, God-given desires. What did you love to play as a child? What could you do for hours on end, without realizing time was passing? There is something so beautifully unfiltered about children—they don't feel the pressure to make money or provide for anyone, and during a certain window, they have zero concern for what other people think about them (even if that means walking out the door in a pajama top, a teal tutu, three different hair accessories, and two different flip-flops!).

I created recipes for fun before I could read and write. I would invite friends over to play "kitchen." This wasn't a Fisher-Price play kitchen—it was our real kitchen! I would keep track of recipes and amounts and times in my head, then ask my mom to write them down and store them forever. When I went to college, this passion continued when I started creating recipes for myself and my friends. This passion has stayed with me all these years, and I still enjoy making recipes for my family and sharing them with other people. I believe there's something about tapping into the magical memories you had as a child that will give you a glimpse into your true desires.

When you think back on your childhood, what were some of your favorite moments? Did you play house? Ride horses? Play outside? Explore in the woods and follow the creek? Play pick-up soccer with neighborhood kids? Paint? How might you be able to follow this passion in adulthood? This doesn't necessarily have to be in the form of a job, but how could you tap into this joy in this stage of your life?

What Makes You Angry about the World?

Frederick Buechner talked about the "world's deep hunger." What is happening in the world that breaks your heart? What is something you wish you could change? What problems keep you awake at night? What injustice strikes righteous anger inside you? What news stories really get you fired up?

To be honest, the fact that there are trillions of problems in the world and I can't fix all of them stresses me out. There are so many things I care about, and I want to see change in all these areas! I get fired up about climate change, healing, fresh-food deserts, and world hunger, to name a few.

One thing to keep in mind when considering this is that God doesn't usually ask us to tackle huge existential problems. We typically start on a small scale, addressing the concerns around us. The problem you're being called to bring justice to might be in your city, your neighborhood, or even within your home.

What Are You Good At?

I might love to play basketball and aspire to be in the WNBA. While that would be amazing, I am five feet two without much athleticism, at least for sports that involve balls and hand-eye coordination. So I can dream as much as I want to, but that future isn't much of a possibility for me. And that's okay! I wasn't made to be a basketball player. If I really loved to play, basketball could be a great hobby for me. It might be a way to meet people, create community, and get some exercise. Or I might find a purpose around basketball that involves supporting other people who play instead of being a professional athlete myself. When thinking of your purpose, try to brainstorm all the ways you naturally excel!

What Are the Pain Points in Your Life?

I have known many people who took their pain and turned it into their purpose. There is something redemptive about going through a difficult circumstance and then helping other people walk through something similar. Having gone through that difficult scenario firsthand, you know what other people need in a powerful and immediate way.

My friend Katie of Wild + Well had a miscarriage, and she now helps women optimize their nutrition to improve their fertility. My friend Carly of Peace Love & Kale received a thyroid cancer diagnosis, and she now helps women pursue healing through clean eating, clean living, and detoxification.

After feeling out of control in terms of my health when I was a child, it was a revelation for me to discover that the food I ate could either make me feel horrible or aid in my healing. This was so freeing for me that I had to tell other people! What once was my pain (literally!) is now the reason I help others.

Is there anything in your life you've been healed from? Anything you've broken free from? Anything you've figured out that you want to share? Leading others to do the same could be part of your purpose.

Finding Your Purpose

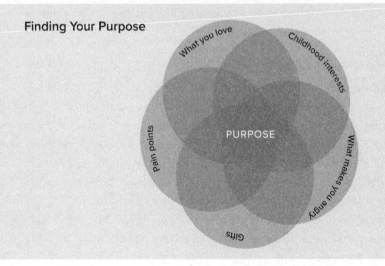

What If Your Purpose Is Your Business?

After you've brainstormed ways to combine your lists, you'll want to determine if your purpose is a volunteer opportunity or a job. While it's wonderful to get paid to do something you love, this is not a requirement. Your job can have meaning even if it's not your life's purpose, and there are ways to fulfill your passions outside of work hours.

If you decide the best combination of your interests, gifts, and desires is to start a business, here are some points to consider. In this chart, you see an example of how to think through your business idea. Let's say you have a ton of ideas, but you're unsure which business you should start first. The first step is to write down all the ideas you are most excited about in the "passion" quadrant.

PASSION	PROFIT
NEED	TIME

Next, rate those ideas based on profit potential. If there are multiple ideas you're equally passionate about but one stands out as a better moneymaker, it makes sense to go with the one you expect to be more profitable and sustainable.

Your next step is to take the top choices from the profit quadrant and filter them through the lens of time. Do you have the time needed to create this business? Is one of your other business ideas less time consuming but potentially equally profitable?

Then put your remaining business ideas through the need filter. Is this solving a real problem for the community you're most passionate about serving? Do people really need the product or service you'd be selling?

Once your chart is filled out, take inventory of your priorities and your life stage. You might have little kiddos at home with no childcare. Your biggest priority might be a business that requires the least time. Or maybe you're ready to quit the corporate world to work on a passion project you've been dreaming about for years. Maybe you have some savings to lean on, so you can prioritize passion over profitability. Regardless of your situation, this chart will help you find out if the business you're dreaming up is the right fit for you right now.

Combine Your Lists

Look back at your lists. What do you love? What did you enjoy as a child? What are you good at? What makes you angry about the world? What are your pain points? Now try to think of ways these lists could intersect. How might your passions meet the world's needs? How could your gifts be used to meet people in their pain? What did you love as a child that could make a difference in the world?

You could even make a Venn diagram that includes each of these categories to help you see how they might overlap. As you're brainstorming how to combine these categories, pay attention to how the options make you feel. If one of them lights you up, that would be a great possibility to explore!

When I look at my lists, I love cooking and food—things I loved as a child too. God has given me gifts in the area of loving people, public speaking, and creativity. When it comes to problems in the world, I am passionate about seeing healing in this world—which includes healing people on this planet and healing the planet. My pain point of feeling unwell as a child led me to help other people find the freedom I experienced. These factors all merged together in the creation of Olive You Whole and in my role as a health coach. Both of these avenues give me the opportunity to help people heal and grow.

Imposter Syndrome

Once you have your idea and you're about to run with it, there's a 100 percent chance you'll bump into a familiar "friend" called imposter syndrome. Imposter syndrome has been described as a sense of self-doubt about our intellect, skills, or accomplishments, especially among high-achieving individuals.[5]

Right now you may be saying to yourself, *Who am I to think I can start this project? Why do I think I have something unique to contribute to the world? I'm not cut out for this—I'll never be able to pull it off.* If that's you, let me encourage you by reminding you that we all have imposter's syndrome at some point.

For the longest time after starting Olive You Whole, I felt like I needed advanced degrees. But Chaz would remind me that I was doing what I wanted to do, which was to create healthy recipes and resources, and people were responding positively. Can you get more education if you want to? Of course! But don't let imposter syndrome stop you from pursuing your dreams.

It's Never Too Late

Just as there's no one right purpose for your life, there's no one right time to start. If something that used to give you meaning starts to feel draining, it may be time to reevaluate and see if your focus needs to shift. You don't need a permission slip to change your mind. You just may be made for more than one amazing purpose!

And if you feel like you're too old to find your purpose and you missed it along the way, I'm here to tell you something: you didn't miss it.

You can choose *today* to do something you're passionate about. If it's been a long time since you felt a calling on your life, or if you've never felt like you were living your purpose, now is the time to make that change, with whatever time you have left on this earth! It will be worth it. As Ichiro Kishimi and Fumitake Koga affirm, "No matter what has occurred in your life up to this point, it should have no bearing at all on how you live from now on. . . You, living in the here and now, are the one who determines your own life."[6]

So take heart! God cares about you so much that he made you uniquely *you*. Only you can fulfill the dream he has created for you! It's fantastic that the things that make our hearts sing he will also use to change the world, one small word or action at a time.

Purpose Challenge

Beginner challenge: Think about something you loved to do as a child. How could you incorporate something similar into your life now? Make it a goal to follow this passion one day a week for a month.

Intermediate challenge: Identify an area you're passionate about, whether it's a volunteer opportunity, a hobby, or a potential job. Find someone who is already engaged in that in some capacity, and ask them to talk with you about what they do and how you might become involved.

Advanced challenge: Meditate on this question: "What do I really want?" Keep digging deeper, asking yourself, *Is that it?* until you feel like you can't ask that question anymore! I want you to think big. Write down your dreams, and try not to filter them too much. Where do you want to be in one year? In two years? In five years? In ten years? Keeping the end in mind helps you stay laser focused as you make more immediate goals.

CONCLUSION

To live is the rarest thing in the world.
Most people exist, that is all.

OSCAR WILDE

A couple of years ago, around Christmas, our daughter, Ella Rae, started getting hives. It began with a few itchy spots on her back and soon became more serious, until she had huge, itchy hives running up her spine and toward her face. Because of the health issues I'd faced as a child, I empathized with what she was going through. But I also felt so empowered.

Her story doesn't have to be my story—now we have tools to help her! After she broke out in hives again and we realized this was a pattern, we knew it was time to tackle the problem. We worked with my health coach, Cynthia Mathes, to find the root cause of Ella Rae's issues. We removed some of the foods that were intolerances for her and focused on healing her gut.

The hives went away, and she felt so much better. While of course I wish she had zero health issues ever, it was healing for me to be able to walk through that experience with her. During her period of healing, she said to me multiple times, "Mommy, I'm so glad you're my mommy and you know how to make me better."

Both Ella Rae's story and my own strengthen my belief that our bodies *want* to heal. God made our bodies to fix, repair, and heal themselves—often in ways that feel miraculous. That's why I wrote this book and why I do the work I do: I want you to fully believe that you can wake up feeling your best every day and live the life of your dreams!

You, my friend, are able to thrive. There are so many tweaks you can make in foundational areas such as food, sleep, movement, rest, and relationships that have a drastic impact on how you feel and how you show up in the world. My hope is that you'll use the tools in this book, one by one, to change your habits to create a life you're proud of.

The improvements you make in your own life impact more than just yourself. Your healthy habits and lifestyle will encourage your children and the people around you to live healthier lives too. You have the opportunity to set them up for a future of flourishing. Little by little, you can make yourself, your home, your family, and the world healthier.

Cheers to your simply healthy life!

DISCUSSION QUESTIONS

These questions can be used on your own to help you go deeper and apply the concepts of each chapter to your life. They can also be used with a friend or with a group as you work through these topics together and hold one another accountable.

Chapter 1: Changing Your Life for Good

1. Do the Magic Wand exercise. If you could wave a magic wand and your life, family, and health could be exactly as you wanted it, what would that look like? Use a stream-of-consciousness style of writing. Don't edit as you go—just write what you're thinking. Try to be as detailed as possible. Where do you live? How do you feel every day? What's your financial situation? What are your relationships like?

2. Of all the things you want to change to create your Magic Wand life, which feels most important or pressing, or which do you feel most passionate about?

3. Craft your answer to the previous question into a SMART goal. Make sure it is specific, measurable, attainable, relevant, and time-bound.

4. What is one good habit you want to develop that's in line with your values and your Magic Wand life? Why do you want to create this habit?

5. What is one bad habit you want to break, and why? Is there a good habit you could replace it with that would fulfill the same reward or desire?

Chapter 2: Food as the Culprit and the Cure

1. Think back to your upbringing as it relates to food. Who influenced your eating habits the most? What experiences impacted the way you eat today?
2. How would you rate your current digestion? Are you experiencing any GI symptoms?
3. How do you navigate the topic of "healthy" and "unhealthy" foods? What do you think about the idea of calling them "all the time" foods and "sometimes" foods? How might a shift in perspective help you handle this tricky topic?
4. What is something you'd like to change about what or how you eat?

Chapter 3: Move Hard, Sleep Hard

1. How would you rate your current level of movement out of 10 (with 0 being barely any movement and 10 being as active as possible)? What factors contribute to that rating?
2. How mobile is your job? If you have a desk job or a job that is very inactive, what are some ways you can move more during the day?
3. Have you ever bought into the lie that exercise should be viewed as a punishment? How do you feel about the idea that movement can bring us joy? Of the types of movement listed, which are you most excited to try?
4. How would you rate your sleep out of 10 (with 0 being very little sleep and 10 being fully rested every night)? Why did you give yourself that rating?
5. What are some ways that you could improve your sleep hygiene?

Chapter 4: The Path to Optimal Functioning

1. Are you experiencing any symptoms that you'd like to find the root cause of? If so, what are they? What steps can you take to find out more?
2. Do you feel like you're getting enough water each day? What could you do to increase your hydration?
3. Take inventory of your personal-care products. Which ones might you choose to investigate or gradually swap out?
4. Look at the list of strategies to support your detoxification system. Which of these ideas would you consider implementing first?
5. For one day, track everything you eat in an app such as MyFitnessPal, and at the end of the day, check your fiber intake. Did you meet the recommended daily fiber target of twenty-five grams per day for women or thirty-eight grams per day for men? If not, what could you add to your eating plan to include more fiber?

Chapter 5: Healthy Home

1. In what ways does your home feel peaceful, like a sanctuary?
2. What are some of your very favorite memories you've made in your current home? What about previous homes?
3. Take inventory of your household cleaning products. Are there any that you could investigate or gradually swap out?
4. Which of the easy swaps described in this chapter would you be interested in trying out in your home? Which do you feel would make the biggest impact?

Chapter 6: Sacred Simplicity

1. In what ways have you believed the lie that more is more?
2. When you think about minimizing, simplifying, and decluttering, what emotions come up for you?

3. Which spaces of your home are most cluttered? Which feel most simple and organized? How do those different spaces make you feel when you're in them?

4. What are your top two personal or family values that will help you know what to say yes to?

5. Which space in your home do you want to simplify first? What's one step you can take to get started?

Chapter 7: Healthy World

1. Consider your commute to work, school, and activities. Are there any strategies for minimizing personal emissions in this chapter that you and your family could try?

2. How could you use your purchasing power to positively impact the planet? Is there something you're considering buying that you could get used?

3. Of the tips for avoiding plastics, which would you like to try? What's one step you could take toward implementing that goal today?

4. When you consider your home energy usage, are there any improvements you could make in this area?

5. When it comes to ways the government can mitigate climate change, which do you feel most excited about? What's one thing you could do to make your voice heard on this topic?

Chapter 8: Building Mental Resilience

1. How would you rank your current mental health out of 10 (with 0 being personal catastrophe and 10 being the best you've ever felt)? Why did you give yourself that rating?

2. What are some of the factors in your life that contribute to your stress? What strategies could you use to mitigate some of the effects of that stress?

3. Of the tools mentioned for managing stress, which one seems like it would be most helpful for your current situation? What's one step you could take to implement that strategy?
4. Which of these struggles has impacted your life: the inner critic, insecurity, judgment, worrying about what other people think, lack of forgiveness, or a victim mentality? In what ways has that struggle affected you? What's one step you could take to be an agent in your own story in this area?

Chapter 9: Finding—and Being—a Good Friend

1. How difficult or easy has it been for you to make friends throughout your life?
2. Are you happy with the number and depth of your friendships? In what ways could your friendships be improved?
3. Are you surprised that friendships are an essential part of good health? Why or why not?
4. Think of a friend you were once close to who you'd like to go deeper with again. What are some ways you can reconnect with them, and how could you maintain that connection? Consider reaching out to them today!

Chapter 10: Harmony at Home

1. What are some of your favorite memories from your family of origin? What is something you loved doing as a child that you could do now as an adult?
2. Take one of the personality tests described in this chapter. What did you learn about yourself?
3. In what ways would it help you to discover more about the personalities of your spouse, children, or other members of your family?
4. How would you rank the communication in your family out

of 10 (with 0 being you're all mimes and 10 being you're the best communicators in the world)? In what ways could your communication improve?

Chapter 11: Sabbath

1. Before reading this chapter, what was your understanding of or experience with the Sabbath?
2. Would you say you're in need of rest? Why or why not?
3. What would you need to do to prepare for a day of Sabbath?
4. Make a list of things you'd like to avoid on your Sabbath. Now make a list of all the things that bring you joy that you'd like to do on the Sabbath.

Chapter 12: Finding Your Purpose

1. In what ways do you currently find purpose in your life?
2. Describe your perfect day. If you could do anything, what would you do?
3. Think about what gets you fired up about what's wrong with our world. How could you become more involved with a solution to that problem?
4. Do you ever struggle with imposter syndrome, like you're not worthy to be doing what you're doing or what you'd like to do? What truth could you tell yourself to fight this mentality?

ACKNOWLEDGMENTS

First and foremost, I have to thank God for giving me the megaphone to write this book. I feel so humbled that being an author is part of my life path!

To my husband, Chaz: you are even more supportive of my work than I knew was possible. Thank you for reading my book and reining in my craziest ideas. I desperately and frequently need you to bring me back down to earth, and you do so with grace. You took on more responsibilities within our family during the busiest seasons of writing and editing, and of course you did so without a single complaint!

To my kiddos: thank you for always encouraging me with your love of my recipes (you are the best taste testers!) and your unlimited supply of hugs, especially when I really need them. You are my biggest, littlest fans.

To everyone who read the long, unedited version of this book or listened to my ideas and provided feedback: I am forever indebted to you! Thank you, Chaz, Mom (Laura Eddleman), Alissa Lozinski, and Katie Braswell. Your insight helped me shape this book, and it shows! I love you so much.

To my agent, Keely Boeving: you are the reason this book exists in the world! I am forever grateful that you believed in me and the message of this book. You are the very best at what you do, and your experience was so helpful as I navigated the nonfiction Christian market for the first time.

To my acquisitions editor at Tyndale, Kara Leonino: I love that you are now both my editor and my friend. Thank you for championing this book. You bring humor and lots of love to everything you do, and you made this process infinitely more enjoyable!

To my editor, Stephanie Rische: I think you had the hardest job of all of us! Thank you for so gracefully squeezing the nearly 120,000 words I submitted into 60,000 in a way that made it feel like nothing was missing! You are brilliant at what you do, and I couldn't have done this without you!

To the Tyndale Refresh team: first of all, thank you for existing. I was so encouraged when I learned that Tyndale had an imprint dedicated to the intersection of faith and wellness. What a gift you are to the world! You are the perfect home for this book.

To my readers and followers: you gave feedback little by little, and you helped me in the writing of this book! Thank you for following, offering support, and making my recipes. You are why I get to wake up every day and why I have the opportunity to do what I do!

MEAL IDEAS

We talked a *lot* about food in chapter 2. It can feel intimidating to go from ideas about nutrition to what's on your plate, so I provided some basic meal ideas you can put together using my general template of protein, greens, vegetables, fat, and optional grain/dairy/extras. Remember: you can get creative and use this template to make an endless variety of meals. Enjoy!

Sushi Bowls

Protein: salmon, tofu, or edamame
Greens: seaweed sheets
Vegetables: carrots, cucumbers
Fat: avocado
Grain: rice
Toppings/Extras: teriyaki sauce, pickled ginger, wasabi

Mediterranean Bowls or Salad

Protein: grilled chicken, chickpeas, or falafel
Greens: salad greens of your choice
Vegetables: cucumbers, tomatoes, red onions, green bell peppers

Fat: kalamata olives
Grain: rice
Dairy: feta cheese
Toppings/Extras: Greek salad dressing, tzatziki sauce, hummus, baba ghanoush

Mexican Bowls, Salad, or Tacos

Protein: ground beef, steak, chicken, pork carnitas, black beans, or pinto beans
Greens: salad greens of your choice
Vegetables: onions, bell peppers
Fat: avocado or guacamole
Grain: corn salsa, tortillas, rice
Dairy: shredded cheese, sour cream
Toppings/Extras: cilantro-lime salad dressing, salsa

Thai Curry Bowls

Protein: chicken breast or tofu
Greens: kale
Vegetables: onions, ginger, garlic, bell peppers, carrots
Fat: coconut oil, coconut milk
Grain: jasmine or basmati rice
Toppings/Extras: Thai red curry paste, lime juice, basil, cilantro

Classic Barbecue

Protein: shredded chicken or pork, beef brisket, baked beans
Greens: coleslaw, kale salad, brussels sprouts
Vegetables: potato salad, cucumber salad
Fat: mayonnaise (in the coleslaw)
Grain: corn on the cob
Toppings/Extras: barbecue sauce, pickles

Classic Southern Meal

Protein: homemade gluten-free fried chicken, catfish, ham,
beef brisket, red beans, or lima beans
Greens: collard greens
Vegetables: sliced tomatoes, green beans, okra, mashed potatoes,
potato salad, wedge fries
Fat: butter
Grain: corn on the cob, grits, cornbread, rice
Toppings/Extras: barbecue sauce, tartar sauce, ketchup

Spanish Paella

Protein: chicken thighs, peas, shrimp, mussels, or calamari
Greens: spinach
Vegetables: scallions, broccoli, artichokes, zucchini, onions,
bell peppers, tomatoes, garlic
Fat: olive oil
Grain: Spanish rice
Toppings/Extras: parsley, saffron, smoked paprika, bay leaves

Minestrone Soup

Protein: chicken or white beans
Greens: spinach
Vegetables: onions, garlic, carrots, zucchini, tomatoes, celery,
green beans
Fat: olive oil, bone broth
Grain: gluten-free pasta
Toppings/Extras: thyme, oregano, rosemary

Eggroll in a Bowl

Protein: ground pork, ground chicken, or tofu
Greens: shredded cabbage
Vegetables: shredded carrots, scallions, garlic, ginger
Fat: sesame oil, cashews
Grain: rice or rice noodles
Toppings/Extras: coconut aminos, cilantro

Stir Fry

Protein: chicken, steak, shrimp, or tofu
Greens: cabbage
Vegetables: onions, bell peppers, carrots, mushrooms, green beans, broccoli, scallions, garlic, ginger
Fat: sesame oil, cashews
Grain: rice or rice noodles
Toppings/Extras: coconut aminos

MENTAL HEALTH RESOURCES

Disaster Distress Helpline: Call or text 1-800-985-5990 to be connected with a trained counselor.

Suicide and Crisis Lifeline: Call or text 988, or chat at 988lifeline.org.

National Domestic Violence Hotline: Call 1-800-799-7233 or text START to 88788.

National Child Abuse Hotline: Call 1-800-4AChild (1-800-422-4453), text 1-800-422-4453, or chat at childhelphotline.org.

National Sexual Assault Hotline: Call 1-800-656-HOPE (4673) or chat at online.rainn.org.

Veterans Crisis Line: Call 988 then press 1, chat at veteranscrisisline .net/get-help-now/chat, or text 838255.

SAMHSA's National Helpline (Substance Abuse and Mental Health Services Administration): Call 1-800-662-HELP (4357).

Treatment Services Locator Website: Go to findahealthcenter.hrsa.gov.

NOTES

CHAPTER 1: CHANGING YOUR LIFE FOR GOOD

1. Duncan Haughey, "A Brief History of SMART Goals," ProjectSmart, December 13, 2014, https://www.projectsmart.co.uk/smart-goals/brief-history-of-smart -goals.php.
2. Natasha Piñon, "Your Key to Success in 2023, Says Attention Expert: The Difference between 'Habits' and 'Routines,'" Make It, CNBC, January 1, 2023, https://www.cnbc.com/2023/01/01/why-everyone-needs-to-know-the-difference -between-habits-and-routines.html.
3. James Clear, *Atomic Habits: An Easy and Proven Way to Build Good Habits and Break Bad Ones* (New York: Avery, 2018).
4. Stacey McLachlan, "The Science of Habit," Healthline, December 22, 2021, https://www.healthline.com/health/the-science-of-habit#1.
5. BJ Fogg, *Tiny Habits: The Small Changes That Change Everything* (New York: Harvest, 2021).
6. James Clear, "Avoid the Second Mistake," James Clear, accessed February 8, 2024, https://jamesclear.com/second-mistake.
7. Jen Sincero, *Badass Habits: Cultivate the Awareness, Boundaries, and Daily Upgrades You Need to Make Them Stick* (New York: Viking, 2020), 30.
8. This exercise was inspired by Fogg, *Tiny Habits*, chap. 2.
9. These habits are adapted from Roxy Vivien, "15 Top Keystone Habits for a Better Year," Roxy Vivien Coaching, January 3, 2022, https://www.roxyvivien .com/15-top-keystone-habits/.
10. Clear, *Atomic Habits*, 54.
11. John Mark Comer, *Practicing the Way: Be with Jesus, Become like Him, Do as He Did* (Colorado Springs: WaterBrook, 2024), 161.

CHAPTER 2: FOOD AS THE CULPRIT AND THE CURE

1. "Disordered Eating and Dieting," National Eating Disorders Collaboration, accessed February 13, 2024, https://nedc.com.au/eating-disorders/eating-disorders-explained/disordered-eating-and-dieting.

2. Tania Strauss, "What Is Regenerative Agriculture and How Can It Help Us Get to Net-Zero Food Systems? 3 Industry Leaders Explain," World Economic Forum, December 19, 2022, https://www.weforum.org/agenda/2022/12/3-industry-leaders-on-achieving-net-zero-goals-with-regenerative-agriculture-practices/; Katy Severson, "Can Meat Actually Save the Planet?" HuffPost, July 18, 2019, https://www.huffpost.com/entry/meat-save-planet-regenerative-farming_l_5d261f7ae4b0583e482b0192.

3. "Why Are CAFOs Bad?," Sierra Club, Michigan Chapter, accessed February 13, 2024, https://www.sierraclub.org/michigan/why-are-cafos-bad.

4. Valerie Baron, "Big Ag Is Hiding in Plain Sight and It's Making Us Sick," National Resources Defense Council, September 23, 2019, https://www.nrdc.org/bio/valerie-baron/big-ag-hiding-plain-sight-and-its-making-us-sick.

5. "Decoding Meat and Dairy Product Labels," Environmental Working Group, accessed February 13, 2024, https://www.ewg.org/research/labeldecoder.

6. Benjamin J. Booth et al., "Livestock and Poultry Density and Childhood Cancer Incidence in Nine States in the USA," *Environmental Research* 159 (November 2017): 444–451, https://www.ncbi.nlm.nih.gov/pmc/articles/PMC5784771/.

7. Strauss, "What Is Regenerative Agriculture?"

8. Juli G. Pausas and Jon E. Keeley, "A Burning Story: The Role of Fire in the History of Life," *BioScience* 59, no. 7 (July 2009): 593–601, https://academic.oup.com/bioscience/article/59/7/593/334816.

9. "Food Label Guide: Seafood," FoodPrint, accessed February 13, 2024, https://foodprint.org/eating-sustainably/food-label-guide/food-label-guide-seafood/.

10. "Understanding 'Certified Sustainable' and the MSC Blue Fish Label," Marine Stewardship Council, accessed February 13, 2024, https://www.msc.org/en-us/what-we-are-doing/our-approach/the-blue-fish-label.

11. Andrew Hazleton, "Difference between Wild Salmon and Wild Caught Salmon," eHow, updated July 25, 2022, https://www.ehow.com/about_6589030_difference-salmon-wild-caught-salmon.html.

12. Amelia Quinn, "Celebrating the Diversity of Chickens and Their Connection to Nature," Greener Ideal, updated January 20, 2024, https://greenerideal.com/news/animals/chicken-diversity-connection-to-nature.

13. Emily Cassidy, "Study: Glyphosate Doubles Risk of Lymphoma," Environmental Working Group, May 23, 2014, https://www.ewg.org/news-insights/news/study-glyphosate-doubles-risk-lymphoma.

14. "Dirty Dozen: EWG's 2023 Shopper's Guide to Pesticides in Produce," Environmental Working Group, https://www.ewg.org/foodnews/dirty-dozen.php.

15. "Clean 15: EWG's 2023 Shopper's Guide to Pesticides in Produce," Environmental Working Group, https://www.ewg.org/foodnews/clean-fifteen.php.

16. Jillian Kubala, "Are Oysters Good for You? Benefits and Dangers," Healthline, June 13, 2023, https://www.healthline.com/nutrition/oysters; Jillian Kubala, "Is Seafood Healthy? Types, Nutrition, Benefits, and Risks," Healthline, https://www.healthline.com/nutrition/is-seafood-healthy.

17. Sarah Ballantyne, "Foundational Foods," Nutrivore, accessed February 13, 2024, https://nutrivore.com/foundational-foods/.

18. Ann F. La Berge, "How the Ideology of Low Fat Conquered America," *Journal of the History of Medicine and Allied Sciences* 63, no. 2 (April 2008): 139–177, https://academic.oup.com/jhmas/article/63/2/139/772615.

19. Chia-Yu Chang, Der-Shin Ke, and Jen-Yin Chen, "Essential Fatty Acids and Human Brain," *Acta Neurologica Taiwanica* 18, no. 4 (December 2009): 231–241, https://pubmed.ncbi.nlm.nih.gov/20329590/.

20. Ruairi Robertson, "What Are the Benefits of Monounsaturated Fats?," Healthline, September 19, 2017, https://www.healthline.com/nutrition/monounsaturated-fats#1.

21. Rajiv Chowdhury et al., "Association of Dietary, Circulating, and Supplement Fatty Acids with Coronary Risk: A Systematic Review and Meta-analysis," *Annals of Internal Medicine* 160, no. 6 (March 18, 2014): 398–406, https://pubmed.ncbi.nlm.nih.gov/24723079/.

22. "Omega-3 Fatty Acids," Cleveland Clinic, last reviewed November 17, 2022, https://my.clevelandclinic.org/health/articles/17290-omega-3-fatty-acids.

23. "Omega-6 Fatty Acids," Mount Sinai, accessed February 13, 2024, https://www.mountsinai.org/health-library/supplement/omega-6-fatty-acids.

24. Tiffany Dobbyn, "Nearly 70% of Private Label Avocado Oil Rancid or Mixed with Other Oils," UC Davis, May 24, 2023, https://www.ucdavis.edu/food/news/70%25-private-label-avocado-oil-rancid-or-mixed-other-oils.

25. Barbara E. Millen et al., "The 2015 Dietary Guidelines Advisory Committee Scientific Report: Development and Major Conclusions," *Advances in Nutrition* 7, no. 3 (May 16, 2016): 438–444, https://pubmed.ncbi.nlm.nih.gov/27184271/.

26. Mark Hyman, *Food: What the Heck Should I Eat?* (New York: Little, Brown, 2018), 68.

27. "Dairy Lobbying," Open Secrets, February 2, 2024, https://www.opensecrets.org/industries/lobbying.php?ind=A04++.

28. "Mandatory Pasteurization for All Milk and Milk Products in Final Package Form Intended for Direct Human Consumption," 21 C.F.R. 1240.61 (as amended December 4, 1992), Code of Federal Regulations, https://www.ecfr.gov/current/title-21/chapter-I/subchapter-L/part-1240/subpart-D/section-1240.61.

29. Eric Berg, "The Fascinating Benefits of Raw Milk Dairy," June 17, 2022, YouTube video, 5:52, https://www.youtube.com/watch?v=PvWz5cNTmLE.

30. "Enzymes," Cleveland Clinic, last reviewed May 12, 2021, https://my.clevelandclinic.org/health/articles/21532-enzymes.

31. *Encyclopedia Britannica*, s.v. "homogenization," April 20, 2021, https://www.britannica.com/science/homogenization.

32. John Lansbury et al., "Relation of the 'Anti-Stiffness Factor' to Collagen Disease and Calcinosis," *Annals of the Rheumatic Diseases* 9, no. 2 (June 1950): 97–108, https://www.ncbi.nlm.nih.gov/pmc/articles/PMC1030753/?page=2.

33. "Lactose Intolerance," Boston Children's Hospital, accessed February 13, 2024, https://www.childrenshospital.org/conditions/lactose-intolerance.

34. "Reports of Selected E. Coli Outbreak Investigations," CDC, last reviewed February 16, 2024, https://www.cdc.gov/ecoli/outbreaks.html.

35. Hyman, *Food*, 205.

36. Alina Petre, "Is Eating Soy Healthy or Unhealthy?," Healthline, August 27, 2020, https://www.healthline.com/nutrition/is-soy-bad-for-you#benefits.

37. A.D.A.M. Medical Encyclopedia, "Healthy Food Trends: Beans and Legumes," MedlinePlus, updated June 22, 2022, https://medlineplus.gov/ency/patientinstructions/000726.htm.

38. Jennifer L. Weinberg, "How to Treat Leptin Resistance: A Functional Medicine Approach," Rupa Health, January 17, 2023, https://www.rupahealth.com/post/how-to-treat-leptin-resistance-a-functional-medicine-approach.

39. "The Sweet Danger of Sugar," Harvard Health Publishing, Harvard Medical School, January 6, 2022, https://www.health.harvard.edu/heart-health/the-sweet-danger-of-sugar.

40. "Artificial Sweeteners and Toxic Side Effects," Dr. Osborne, accessed February 12, 2024, https://www.drpeterosborne.com/artificial-sweeteners-toxic-side-effects/.

41. Christina R. Whitehouse, Joseph Boullata, and Linda A. McCauley, "The Potential Toxicity of Artificial Sweeteners," *AAOHN Journal* 56, no. 6 (June 2008): 251–259, https://pubmed.ncbi.nlm.nih.gov/18604921/.

42. Helen West, "Do Artificial Sweeteners Spike Your Blood Sugar?," Healthline, June 3, 2017, https://www.healthline.com/nutrition/artificial-sweeteners-blood-sugar-insulin.

43. Corey Whelan, "Honey vs. Sugar: Which Sweetener Should I Use?," Healthline, updated May 19, 2023, https://www.healthline.com/health/food-nutrition/honey-vs-sugar; Kristin Kirkpatrick, "Is Maple Syrup Better for You Than Sugar?," Cleveland Clinic, September 21, 2021, https://health.clevelandclinic.org/is-maple-syrup-better-for-you-than-sugar; Laren Panoff, "Is Coconut Sugar a Nutritious Replacement?," updated December 12, 2023, https://www.verywellhealth.com/coconut-sugar-8407729.

44. Sanjay Gupta, "If We Are What We Eat, Americans Are Corn and Soy," CNN Health, September 22, 2007, https://www.cnn.com/2007/HEALTH/diet.fitness/09/22/kd.gupta.column/.

45. Tanya L. Blasbalg et al., "Changes in Consumption of Omega-3 and Omega-6 Fatty Acids in the United States during the 20th Century," *American Journal of Clinical Nutrition* 93, no. 5 (May 2011): 950–962, https://www.ncbi.nlm.nih.gov/pmc/articles/PMC3076650.

46. "Inflammation," Cleveland Clinic, last reviewed December 20, 2023, https://my.clevelandclinic.org/health/symptoms/21660-inflammation.

NOTES

47. "Artificial Trans Fats Banned in US," Harvard T. H. Chan School of Public Health, https://www.hsph.harvard.edu/news/hsph-in-the-news/us-bans-artificial-trans-fats/.
48. Sarah Rehkamp, "A Look at Calorie Sources in the American Diet," Economic Research Service, U.S. Department of Agriculture, December 5, 2016, https://www.ers.usda.gov/amber-waves/2016/december/a-look-at-calorie-sources-in-the-american-diet.
49. Hyman, *Food*, 188.
50. Melanie Uhde et al., "Intestinal Cell Damage and Systemic Immune Activation in Individuals Reporting Sensitivity to Wheat in the Absence of Coeliac Disease," *Gut* 65, no. 12 (December 2016): 1930–1937, https://pubmed.ncbi.nlm.nih.gov/27459152.
51. Intersalt Cooperative Research Group, "Intersalt: An International Study of Electrolyte Excretion and Blood Pressure. Results for 24 Hour Urinary Sodium and Potassium Excretion," *BMJ* 297, no. 6644 (July 30, 1988): 319–328, https://pubmed.ncbi.nlm.nih.gov/3416162.
52. "The Nutrition Source: Healthy Eating Plate vs. USDA's MyPlate," Harvard T.H. Chan School of Public Health, last reviewed February 2023, https://www.hsph.harvard.edu/nutritionsource/healthy-eating-plate-vs-usda-myplate.
53. "The Fab Four," Be Well, accessed February 12, 2024, https://bewellbykelly.com/pages/fab-four.

CHAPTER 3: MOVE HARD, SLEEP HARD

1. "Exercising for Better Sleep," Johns Hopkins Medicine, accessed February 8, 2024, https://www.hopkinsmedicine.org/health/wellness-and-prevention/exercising-for-better-sleep.
2. "The Women's League of Health and Beauty: Nazis, Pilates and the Birth of the Keep-Fit Movement," Flashbak, March 8, 2014, https://flashbak.com/the-womens-league-of-health-and-beauty-nazis-pilates-and-the-birth-of-the-keep-fit-movement-4580/.
3. Natalia Mehlman Petrzela, *Fit Nation: The Gains and Pains of America's Exercise Obsession* (Chicago: University of Chicago Press, 2022), 203–204.
4. "Workouts through History," Health Life, March 1, 2019, https://healthlifemagazine.com/2019/03/01/workouts-through-history.
5. Luke C. Strotz et al., "Metabolic Rates, Climate and Macroevolution: A Case Study Using Neogene Molluscs," *Proceedings of the Royal Society B* 285, no. 1885 (August 22, 2018), https://royalsocietypublishing.org/doi/10.1098/rspb.2018.1292; "People Prefer Being Lazy Because Our Brains Are Wired That Way, Study Says," CBC, September 18, 2018, https://www.cbc.ca/news/canada/british-columbia/our-brains-are-hardwired-for-laziness-ubc-study-shows-1.4828474.
6. "Occupational Requirements Survey," U.S. Bureau of Labor Statistics, accessed February 8, 2024, https://www.bls.gov/ors/latest-numbers.htm.

7. "How Much Physical Activity Do Adults Need?," Centers for Disease Control and Prevention, June 2, 2022, https://www.cdc.gov/physicalactivity/basics/adults/index.htm.

8. "Benefits of Physical Activity," Centers for Disease Control and Prevention, August 1, 2023, https://www.cdc.gov/physicalactivity/basics/pa-health/index.htm.

9. "Benefits of Physical Activity," Centers for Disease Control and Prevention.

10. "Lymphatic System," Better Health Channel, July 19, 2017, https://www.betterhealth.vic.gov.au/health/conditionsandtreatments/lymphatic-system; Roxana Ehsani, "Does Exercise Improve Your Immune System? Here's What the Research Says," *EatingWell*, November 3, 2023, https://www.eatingwell.com/does-exercise-improve-your-immune-system-8386750#.

11. "Exercising to Relax," Harvard Health Publishing, July 7, 2020, https://www.health.harvard.edu/staying-healthy/exercising-to-relax.

12. Michael Gleeson et al., "The Anti-Inflammatory Effects of Exercise: Mechanisms and Implications for the Prevention and Treatment of Disease," *Nature Reviews Immunology* 11 (2011): 607–615, https://www.nature.com/articles/nri3041.

13. Robby Berman, "Is Exercise More Effective Than Medication for Depression and Anxiety?," Medical News Today, March 3, 2023, https://www.medicalnewstoday.com/articles/is-exercise-more-effective-than-medication-for-depression-and-anxiety.

14. Berman, "Is Exercise More Effective Than Medication for Depression and Anxiety?"

15. Amy Kreger, "Definition of Cardio Exercise," Livestrong.com, accessed February 8, 2024, https://www.livestrong.com/article/114986-definition-cardio-exercise/.

16. "Aerobic Exercise: Top 10 Reasons to Get Physical," Mayo Clinic, November 18, 2023, https://www.mayoclinic.org/healthy-lifestyle/fitness/in-depth/aerobic-exercise/art-20045541.

17. Thitiporn Supasitthumrong, "Endorphins: The 'Feel Good' Chemicals for Well-Being," MedPark Hospital, July 31, 2023, https://www.medparkhospital.com/en-US/lifestyles/endorphins.

18. "Walking for Good Health," Better Health Channel, February 20, 2023, https://www.betterhealth.vic.gov.au/health/healthyliving/walking-for-good-health.

19. Alex Hutchinson, "Is Group Exercise Better Than Working Out Solo?," *Globe and Mail*, January 6, 2010, https://www.theglobeandmail.com/life/health-and-fitness/fitness/is-group-exercise-better-than-working-out-solo/article4268232/.

20. Katey Davidson, "14 Benefits of Strength Training," Healthline, August 16, 2021, https://www.healthline.com/health/fitness/benefits-of-strength-training#bottom-line.

21. "Stretching: Focus on Flexibility," Mayo Clinic, November 18, 2023, https://www.mayoclinic.org/healthy-lifestyle/fitness/in-depth/stretching/art-20047931.

22. I've met some Christians who have objections to doing yoga because of its Hindu and Buddhist roots. I agree that everything we do should be done with discernment. When I think about yoga, I am reminded of James 1:17: "Every good and perfect gift is from above." The physical movements found in yoga can

be beneficial for my body, and when applied thoughtfully, these movements and breath work can improve both physical and emotional wellness.

23. Susan L. Worley, "The Extraordinary Importance of Sleep: The Detrimental Effects of Inadequate Sleep on Health and Public Safety Drive an Explosion of Sleep Research," *Pharmacy and Therapeutics* 43, no. 12 (December 2018): 758–763, https://www.ncbi.nlm.nih.gov/pmc/articles/PMC6281147/.

24. Kirsten Nunez and Karen Lamoreux, "What Is the Purpose of Sleep?," Healthline, June 20, 2023, https://www.healthline.com/health/why-do-we-sleep.

25. "Convention against Torture and Other Cruel, Inhuman or Degrading Treatment or Punishment," Senate Consideration of Treaty Document 100-20, Congress.gov, April 18, 1988, https://www.congress.gov/treaty-document/100th-congress/20/resolution-text.

26. Kelly Bulkeley, "Why Sleep Deprivation Is Torture," *Psychology Today*, December 15, 2014, https://www.psychologytoday.com/us/blog/dreaming-in-the-digital-age/201412/why-sleep-deprivation-is-torture.

27. Bulkeley, "Why Sleep Deprivation Is Torture."

28. Worley, "Extraordinary Importance of Sleep."

29. "How Much Sleep Do I Need?," Centers for Disease Control and Prevention, September 14, 2022, https://www.cdc.gov/sleep/about_sleep/how_much_sleep.html.

30. Eric Suni and Abhinav Singh, "How Much Sleep Do You Need?," Sleep Foundation, January 3, 2024, https://www.sleepfoundation.org/how-sleep-works/how-much-sleep-do-we-really-need.

31. Manar Al Kazhali et al., "Social Media Use Is Linked to Poor Sleep Quality: The Opportunities and Challenges to Support Evidence-Informed Policymaking in the UAE," *Journal of Public Health* 45, no. 1 (March 14, 2023): 124–133, https://pubmed.ncbi.nlm.nih.gov/34693449.

32. Kazhali, "Social Media Use Is Linked to Poor Sleep Quality."

33. Jay Rai, "Why You Should Stop Checking Your Phone in the Morning (and What to Do Instead)," *Forbes*, April 2, 2021, https://www.forbes.com/sites/forbescoachescouncil/2021/04/02/why-you-should-stop-checking-your-phone-in-the-morning-and-what-to-do-instead/?sh=6ff743572684.

34. "Insomnia," Cleveland Clinic, February 13, 2023, https://my.clevelandclinic.org/health/diseases/12119-insomnia.

35. "Circadian Rhythms," National Institute of General Medical Sciences, September 2023, https://nigms.nih.gov/education/fact-sheets/Pages/circadian-rhythms.aspx.

36. "Circadian Rhythms."

CHAPTER 4: THE PATH TO OPTIMAL FUNCTIONING

1. "The Importance of Hydration," Harvard T.H. Chan School of Public Health, accessed February 18, 2024, https://www.hsph.harvard.edu/news/hsph-in-the-news/the-importance-of-hydration; Kathleen Zelman, "6 Reasons to Drink

Water," WebMD, April 4, 2022, https://www.webmd.com/diet/features/6-reasons
-to-drink-water.

2. Sara Shriber, "Forty-Seven Percent of Americans Don't Drink Enough Water,
Plus More Water Insights," Civic Science, January 17, 2023, https://civicscience
.com/forty-seven-percent-of-americans-dont-drink-enough-water-plus-more
-h2o-insights/.

3. Barry M. Popkin, Kristen E. D'Anci, and Irwin H. Rosenberg, "Water, Hydration
and Health," *Nutrition Reviews* 68, no. 8 (August 1, 2010): 439–458, https://
academic.oup.com/nutritionreviews/article/68/8/439/1841926.

4. Yanan Wang, "In Flint, Mich., There's So Much Lead in Children's Blood That a
State of Emergency Is Declared," *Washington Post*, December 15, 2015, https://
www.washingtonpost.com/news/morning-mix/wp/2015/12/15/toxic-water-soaring
-lead-levels-in-childrens-blood-create-state-of-emergency-in-flint-mich.

5. Cecilia Reyes and Michael Hawthorne, "Brain-Damaging Lead Found in Tap
Water in Hundreds of Homes Tested across Chicago, Results Show," *Chicago
Tribune*, April 12, 2018, https://www.chicagotribune.com/investigations/ct
-chicago-water-lead-contamination-20180411-htmlstory.html.

6. "Consumer Confidence Reports (CCR)," United States Environmental Protection
Agency, accessed February 18, 2024, https://ordspub.epa.gov/ords/safewater/f?p
=ccr_wyl:102.

7. "EWG's Tap Water Database," Environmental Working Group, accessed February
18, 2024, https://www.ewg.org/tapwater/.

8. "Bottled Water Everywhere: Keeping It Safe," U.S. Food and Drug Administration,
April 22, 2022, https://www.fda.gov/consumers/consumer-updates/bottled-water
-everywhere-keeping-it-safe.

9. Matthew Boesler, "Bottled Water Costs 2000 Times as Much as Tap Water,"
Business Insider, July 12, 2013, https://www.businessinsider.com/bottled-water
-costs-2000x-more-than-tap-2013-7.

10. "Men's Use of Personal Care Products Has Doubled Since 2004, according
to New Consumer Survey," Environmental Working Group, July 26, 2023,
https://www.ewg.org/news-insights/news-release/2023/07/mens-use-personal
-care-products-has-doubled-2004-according-new.

11. Homer Swei et al., "Survey Finds Use of Personal Care Products Up Since 2004:
What That Means for Your Health," Environmental Working Group, July 26,
2023, https://www.ewg.org/research/survey-finds-use-personal-care-products
-2004-what-means-your-health.

12. "Unacceptable List: Personal Care Products," EWG Verified, accessed March 8,
2024, chrome-extension://efaidnbmnnnibpcajpcglclefindmkaj/https://static.ewg
.org/upload/pdf/EWGV_Lists_PCP-No.pdf?_ga=2.118941390.652678959
.1708311009-1546709908.1707453650.

13. "Understanding Skin Deep Ratings," EWG's Skin Deep, Environmental
Working Group, accessed February 19, 2024, https://www.ewg.org/skindeep
/understanding_skin_deep_ratings/.

NOTES

14. "Constipation," Health, Johns Hopkins Medicine, accessed February 19, 2024, https://www.hopkinsmedicine.org/health/conditions-and-diseases/constipation.

15. Charlie Wettlaufer, "Calculating Food Costs for Cold Pressed Juice," Goodnature, September 2, 2014, https://www.goodnature.com/blog/calculating-food-costs-for-cold-pressed-juice.

16. Taylor Jones and Rachael Ajmera, "11 Foods That Are Good for Your Liver," Healthline, updated October 30, 2023, https://www.healthline.com/nutrition/11-foods-for-your-liver.

17. Millie Lytle, "A New Way to Detox: Eat to Support 6 Organs of Elimination," mindbodygreen, July 27, 2023, https://www.mindbodygreen.com/articles/what-to-eat-to-support-your-6-organs-of-elimination.

18. Naghma Khan and Hasan Mukhtar, "Tea and Health: Studies in Humans," *Current Pharmaceutical Design*, June 12, 2014, https://www.ncbi.nlm.nih.gov/pmc/articles/PMC4055352.

19. Tudor Andrei Cernomaz, Sorin Gheorghe Bolog, and Traian Mihăescu, "The Effect of a Dry Salt Inhaler in Adults with COPD," *Pneumologia* 56, no. 3 (July–September 2007): 124–127, https://pubmed.ncbi.nlm.nih.gov/18019972/.

20. "Is Rinsing Your Sinuses with Neti Pots Safe?," U.S. Food and Drug Administration, October 5, 2023, https://www.fda.gov/consumers/consumer-updates/rinsing-your-sinuses-neti-pots-safe.

21. Gerry K. Schwalfenberg, "The Alkaline Diet: Is There Evidence That an Alkaline pH Diet Benefits Health?," *Journal of Environmental and Public Health* 2012 (October 12, 2011): 727630, https://www.ncbi.nlm.nih.gov/pmc/articles/PMC3195546/.

22. Ronni Gordon, "The Benefits and Risks of Dry Brushing," Healthline, updated March 14, 2023, https://www.healthline.com/health/dry-brushing.

23. Margaret E. Sears, Kathleen J. Kerr, Riina I. Bray, "Arsenic, Cadmium, Lead, and Mercury in Sweat: A Systematic Review," Journal of Environmental Public Health, https://www.ncbi.nlm.nih.gov/pmc/articles/PMC3312275/.

24. "Alternative Cancer Treatments," Hope4Cancer, accessed February 19, 2024, https://hope4cancer.com/alternative-cancer-treatments/.

25. Julia Belluz, "Nearly All Americans Fail to Eat Enough of This Actual Superfood," Vox, July 15, 2019, https://www.vox.com/2019/3/20/18214505/fiber-diet-weight-loss.

26. "Dietary Fiber: Essential for a Healthy Diet," Mayo Clinic, November 4, 2022, https://www.mayoclinic.org/healthy-lifestyle/nutrition-and-healthy-eating/in-depth/fiber/art-20043983.

27. Belluz, "Nearly All Americans."

28. "Dietary Fiber," Mayo Clinic.

29. Joe Leech, "Fiber Can Help You Lose Weight—But Only a Specific Type," Healthline, updated February 8, 2023, https://www.healthline.com/nutrition/fiber-can-help-you-lose-weight.

30. Dorothy A. Kieffer, Roy J. Martin, and Sean H. Adams, "Impact of Dietary Fibers

on Nutrient Management and Detoxification Organs: Gut, Liver, and Kidneys," *Advances in Nutrition* 7, no. 6 (November 2016): 1111–1121, https://www.ncbi .nlm.nih.gov/pmc/articles/PMC5105045/.

31. Jillian Levy, "Top 25 Insoluble Fiber Foods and Surprising Benefits beyond Constipation Relief," Dr. Axe, July 12, 2023, https://draxe.com/nutrition /insoluble-fiber/.

32. Yuhui Li et al., "Wheat Bran Intake Can Attenuate Chronic Cadmium Toxicity in Mice Gut Microbiota," *Food and Function* 7, no. 8 (August 10, 2016): 3524–3530, https://pubmed.ncbi.nlm.nih.gov/27425201/.

33. Sharon O'Brien, "Top 20 Foods High in Soluble Fiber," Healthline, updated January 11, 2024, https://www.healthline.com/nutrition/foods-high-in -soluble-fiber.

34. Levy, "Top 25 Insoluble Fiber Foods."

CHAPTER 5: HEALTHY HOME

1. "Why Indoor Air Quality Is Important to Schools," United States Environmental Protection Agency, November 28, 2023, https://www.epa.gov/iaq-schools/why -indoor-air-quality-important-schools.

2. "Exposure and Health Effects of Chemicals," Government of Canada, August 23, 2023, https://www.canada.ca/en/health-canada/services/health-effects-chemical -exposure.html.

3. "Indoor Air Quality," United States Environmental Protection Agency.

4. "Exposure and Health Effects of Chemicals," Government of Canada.

5. "Indoor Air Quality," United States Environmental Protection Agency.

6. "Indoor Air Quality," United States Environmental Protection Agency.

7. "Frequently Asked Questions on Safer Choice," United States Environmental Protection Agency, November 15, 2023, https://www.epa.gov/saferchoice /frequently-asked-questions-safer-choice.

8. "About EWG's Guide to Healthy Cleaning," Environmental Working Group, accessed February 16, 2024, https://www.ewg.org/guides/cleaners/content /methodology/.

9. "Household Cleaner Ratings and Ingredients," Environmental Working Group, accessed February 16, 2024, https://www.ewg.org/guides/cleaners/content /findings/.

10. Samara Geller, "Skip the Most Toxic Fabric Softeners," Environmental Working Group, August 16, 2022, https://www.ewg.org/news-insights/news/2022/08 /skip-most-toxic-fabric-softeners.

11. "About EWG's Guide to Healthy Cleaning," Environmental Working Group.

12. "What Are Volatile Organic Compounds (VOCs)?," United States Environmental Protection Agency, March 15, 2023, https://www.epa.gov/indoor-air-quality-iaq /what-are-volatile-organic-compounds-vocs.

13. Robert Coleman, "EWG News Roundup (10/2): California Cosmetics Bill Signed into Law, Algae Beach Closures and More," Environmental Working

Group, October 2, 2020, https://www.ewg.org/news-insights/news/ewg-news-roundup-102-california-cosmetics-bill-signed-law-algae-beach-closures.

14. "What Is BPA, and Where Is It Found?," Environmental Working Group, accessed February 16, 2024, https://www.ewg.org/areas-focus/toxic-chemicals/bpa.

15. "What Is BPA, and Where Is It Found?," Environmental Working Group.

16. Tammy Zhao, "What's in Drain Cleaner, and What Happens if You Drink It?," Poison Control, accessed February 16, 2024, https://www.poison.org/articles/whats-in-drain-cleaner.

17. "Household Cleaner Ratings and Ingredients," Environmental Working Group.

18. "About EWG's Guide to Healthy Cleaning," Environmental Working Group.

19. "FAQs: Candles," Children's Environmental Health Network, accessed February 16, 2024, https://cehn.org/our-work/eco-healthy-child-care/ehcc-faqs/candles/.

20. B. C. Wolverton, Anne Johnson, and Keith Bounds, "Interior Landscape Plants for Indoor Air Pollution Abatement," NASA, September 15, 1989, https://ntrs.nasa.gov/citations/19930073077; Dana Nichols, "The Best Plants to Help Purify the Air in Your Home," House Digest, December 6, 2022, https://www.housedigest.com/1128572/the-best-plants-to-help-purify-the-air-in-your-home/.

21. Erica Cirino and Karen Lamoreux, "Should You Be Worried about EMF Exposure?," Healthline, December 8, 2023, https://www.healthline.com/health/emf.

CHAPTER 6: SACRED SIMPLICITY

1. Jordan T. Prodanoff, "How Many Ads Do We See a Day? 17 Insightful Stats," Web Tribunal, March 6, 2023, https://webtribunal.net/blog/how-many-ads-do-we-see-a-day/.

2. "Advertising Spending in North America from 2000 to 2024," Statista, September 19, 2023, https://www.statista.com/statistics/429036/advertising-expenditure-in-north-america/.

3. Carmen Ang, "The Median Home Size in Every U.S. State in 2022," Visual Capitalist, November 22, 2022, https://www.visualcapitalist.com/cp/median-home-size-every-american-state-2022.

4. Alan Bernau Jr., "54 Self-Storage Industry Statistics You Should Know for 2023," Alan's Factory Outlet, updated October 20, 2023, https://alansfactoryoutlet.com/blog/self-storage-industry-statistics/.

5. I absolutely love Brené Brown's values exercise. Find out more at https://brenebrown.com/resources/living-into-our-values/.

6. Lauren Silva, "The Mental Health Benefits of a Clean Home," Forbes Health, *Forbes*, December 1, 2022, https://www.forbes.com/health/mind/mental-health-clean-home/.

7. Ellen Chang, "How Long Should You Keep Tax Records?," Forbes Advisor, *Forbes*, October 28, 2022, https://www.forbes.com/advisor/taxes/how-long-do-you-keep-tax-records.

8. Pixie Technology, "Lost and Found: The Average American Spends 2.5 Days Each Year Looking for Lost Items Collectively Costing U.S. Households

$2.7 Billion Annually in Replacement Costs," PR Newswire, May 2, 2017, https://www.prnewswire.com/news-releases/lost-and-found-the-average-american -spends-25-days-each-year-looking-for-lost-items-collectively-costing-us -households-27-billion-annually-in-replacement-costs-300449305.html.

9. Marie Kondo, *The Life-Changing Magic of Tidying Up: The Japanese Art of Decluttering and Organizing,* trans. Cathy Hirano (Berkeley: Ten Speed Press, 2014), 153–154.

10. Kent Nerburn, *Simple Truths: Clear and Gentle Guidance on the Big Issues in Life* (Novato, CA: New World Library, 2019), 44.

CHAPTER 7: HEALTHY WORLD

1. Brian Bushard, "What Is the Anthropocene Epoch—and Why Do Scientists Think a Lake in Suburban Canada Defines It?," *Forbes,* July 11, 2023, https:// www.forbes.com/sites/brianbushard/2023/07/11/what-is-the-anthropocene -epoch-and-why-do-scientists-think-a-lake-in-suburban-canada-defines-it/?sh =4a79698247ad.

2. Daniel Politi, "U.N. Panel Warns World Only Has 12 Years to Avert Climate Change Crisis," Slate, October 8, 2018, https://slate.com/news-and-politics /2018/10/un-intergovernmental-panel-on-climate-change-ipcc-warns-world -only-has-12-years-to-avert-climate-change-crisis.html.

3. Nathan Rott, "Extreme Weather, Fueled by Climate Change, Cost the U.S. $165 Billion in 2022," *All Things Considered,* NPR, January 10, 2023, https:// www.npr.org/2023/01/10/1147986096/extreme-weather-fueled-by-climate -change-cost-the-u-s-165-billion-in-2022.

4. Anne Makovec and Molly McCrea, "Farmer Shows Path Forward as California Composting Law Goes into Effect," CBS News, August 17, 2023, https:// www.cbsnews.com/sanfrancisco/news/project-earth-cultivating-compost -california-crop.

5. "Zero Waste Case Study: San Francisco," United States Environmental Protection Agency, updated November 22, 2023, https://www.epa.gov/transforming-waste -tool/zero-waste-case-study-san-francisco.

6. Anne Makovec and Molly McCrea, "Farmer Shows Path Forward as California Composting Law Goes into Effect," CBS News, August 17, 2023, https:// www.cbsnews.com/sanfrancisco/news/project-earth-cultivating-compost -california-crop/.

7. "Cooler Smarter: Geek Out on the Data!," Union of Concerned Scientists, March 29, 2012, https://www.ucsusa.org/resources/cooler-smarter-geek -out-data.

8. "Cooler Smarter," Union of Concerned Scientists.

9. "Calculate Your Carbon Footprint," Nature Conservancy, accessed February 19, 2024, https://www.nature.org/en-us/get-involved/how-to-help/carbon-footprint -calculator/.

10. "Transportation," Union of Concerned Scientists, accessed February 19, 2024, https://www.ucsusa.org/transportation.
11. "Greenest: Model Year 2023," Greenercars.org, accessed February 20, 2024, https://greenercars.org/greenest-meanest/greenest.
12. Melissa Denchak, "How You Can Stop Global Warming," Natural Resources Defense Council (NRDC), August 7, 2023, https://www.nrdc.org/stories/how-you-can-stop-global-warming.
13. Jack Flynn, "15+ Average Commute Time Statistics [2023]: How Long Is the Average American Commute?," Zippia, February 13, 2023, https://www.zippia.com/advice/average-commute-time-statistics/.
14. "Fossil Fuels and Plastic," Center for International Environmental Law, accessed February 20, 2024, https://www.ciel.org/issue/fossil-fuels-plastic/.
15. Steph Coelho, "What Temperature Should I Set My Thermostat in Winter?," Bob Vila, updated January 29, 2024, https://www.bobvila.com/articles/what-temperature-should-i-set-my-thermostat-in-winter/.
16. "Cooler Smarter," Union of Concerned Scientists.
17. "Air Sealing Your Home," Office of Energy Saver, U.S. Department of Energy, accessed February 20, 2024, https://www.energy.gov/energysaver/air-sealing-your-home.
18. "Energy Efficient Products for Consumers," Energy Star, accessed February 20, 2024, https://www.energystar.gov/products.
19. "Tips for Managing Your Electric Usage," New Hampshire Department of Energy, accessed February 20, 2024, https://www.energy.nh.gov/consumers/energy-efficiency/energy-efficiency-programs-and-services/tips-managing-your-electric.
20. Scott Minos, "3 Easy Tips to Reduce Your Standby Power Loads," Office of Energy Saver, U.S. Department of Energy, February 9, 2022, https://www.energy.gov/energysaver/articles/3-easy-tips-reduce-your-standby-power-loads.
21. G. E. Miller, "Stop Wasting Money on Electricity! A Guide to Identifying and Unplugging Standby Power Appliances," 20somethingfinance, updated January 3, 2024, https://20somethingfinance.com/electrical-leaking-standby-appliance-list/.
22. "Wireless Devices: Potential Cancer Risk Says World Health Organization," EMF Safety Network, May 31, 2011, http://emfsafetynetwork.org/wireless-devices-potential-cancer-risk-says-world-health-organization/.
23. "Lighting Choices to Save You Money," Office of Energy Saver, U.S. Department of Energy, accessed February 20, 2024, https://www.energy.gov/energysaver/lighting-choices-save-you-money.
24. Nafeesah Allen and Corinne Tynan, "How Much Power Does a Solar Panel Produce?," *Forbes*, updated August 1, 2023, https://www.forbes.com/home-improvement/solar/how-much-power-does-a-solar-panel-produce/.
25. Chauncey Crail and Corinne Tynan, "How Much Do Solar Panels Save the Average Homeowner?," *Forbes*, updated July 28, 2023, https://www.forbes.com/home-improvement/solar/how-much-solar-panels-save/.
26. "10 Ways to Save Water at Home," American Rivers, accessed February 20,

2024, https://www.americanrivers.org/rivers/discover-your-river/top-10-ways
-for-you-to-save-water-at-home/; "25 Ways to Save Water," Volusia County
Florida, accessed February 20, 2024, https://www.volusia.org/services/growth
-and-resource-management/environmental-management/natural-resources/water
-conservation/25-ways-to-save-water.stml.

27. "How Do Governments Combat Climate Change?," World101, updated July
25, 2023, https://world101.cfr.org/global-era-issues/climate-change/how-do
-governments-combat-climate-change.
28. "Air Pollution," World Health Organization, accessed February 20, 2024,
https://www.who.int/health-topics/air-pollution#tab=tab_2.
29. "USA Funds Nuclear-Coupled Carbon Capture Studies," World Nuclear News
(WNN), April 21, 2022, https://world-nuclear-news.org/Articles/USA-funds
-nuclear-coupled-carbon-capture-studies.

CHAPTER 8: BUILDING MENTAL RESILIENCE
1. "About Mental Health," Centers for Disease Control and Prevention, last
reviewed April 25, 2023, https://www.cdc.gov/mentalhealth/learn/index.htm.
2. "Mental Illness," National Institute of Mental Health, updated March 2023,
https://www.nimh.nih.gov/health/statistics/mental-illness.
3. "What's the Difference between Stress and Anxiety?," American Psychological
Association, updated February 14, 2022, https://www.apa.org/topics/stress
/anxiety-difference.
4. "Stress," World Health Organization, February 21, 2023, https://www.who.int
/news-room/questions-and-answers/item/stress.
5. Martin Taylor, "What Does Fight, Flight, Freeze, Fawn Mean?," WebMD, April
28, 2022, https://www.webmd.com/mental-health/what-does-fight-flight-freeze
-fawn-mean.
6. Avi Solomon, "Stanford's Prof. Robert Sapolsky on Coping with Stress: An
Interview," Learning for Life, Medium, September 1, 2014, https://medium
.com/learning-for-life/robert-sapolsky-on-stress-an-interview-c7e372e2f68e.
7. Yun-Zi Liu, Yun-Xia Wang, and Chun-Lei Jiang, "Inflammation: The Common
Pathway of Stress-Related Diseases," *Frontiers in Human Neuroscience* 11 (June
20, 2017): 316, https://www.ncbi.nlm.nih.gov/pmc/articles/PMC5476783.
8. "Stress Effects on the Body," American Psychological Association, last updated
March 8, 2023, https://www.apa.org/topics/stress/body.
9. "Stress Effects on the Body," American Psychological Association.
10. "Chronic Stress Puts Your Health at Risk," Mayo Clinic, August 1, 2023,
https://www.mayoclinic.org/healthy-lifestyle/stress-management/in-depth
/stress/art-20046037.
11. "Chronic Stress," Yale Medicine, accessed February 21, 2024, https://
www.yalemedicine.org/conditions/stress-disorder.
12. Solomon, "Stanford's Prof. Robert Sapolsky on Coping with Stress."
13. Abiola Keller et al., "Does the Perception That Stress Affects Health Matter?

The Association with Health and Mortality," *Health Psychology* 31, no. 5 (September 2012): 677–684, https://www.ncbi.nlm.nih.gov/pmc/articles /PMC3374921/.

14. Keller et al., "Does the Perception That Stress Affects Health Matter?"
15. Andrew L. Geers et al., "Further Evidence for Individual Differences in Placebo Responding: An Interactionist Perspective," *Journal of Psychosomatic Research* 62, no. 5 (May 2007): 563–570, https://pubmed.ncbi.nlm.nih.gov/17467411/; Toshihiko Maruta et al., "Optimism-Pessimism Assessed in the 1960s and Self-Reported Health Status 30 Years Later," *Mayo Clinic Proceedings* 77, no. 8 (August 2002): 748–753, https://pubmed.ncbi.nlm.nih.gov/12173709/.
16. Jennifer J. Heisz, *Move the Body, Heal the Mind: Overcome Anxiety, Depression, and Dementia and Improve Focus, Creativity, and Sleep* (Boston: Mariner Books, 2022).
17. Emma M. Seppälä et al., "Promoting Mental Health and Psychological Thriving in University Students: A Randomized Controlled Trial of Three Well-Being Interventions," *Frontiers in Psychiatry* 11 (July 15, 2020): 590, https://www .frontiersin.org/articles/10.3389/fpsyt.2020.00590/full.
18. Karthik Kumar, "Why Do Navy SEALs Use Box Breathing?" MedicineNet, accessed February 22, 2024, https://www.medicinenet.com/why_do_navy_seals _use_box_breathing/article.htm.
19. Thanks to yoga instructor Rachel Brathen for this terminology.
20. Ichiro Kishimi and Fumitake Koga, *The Courage to Be Disliked* (London: Allen and Unwin, 2019), 140–141.
21. Hadley Vlahos (@nurse.hadley), "Top Three Regrets at the End of Life," Instagram, May 3, 2023, https://www.instagram.com/p/Cryr3TtJj0E/?hl=en.
22. Man Yee Ho et al., "International REACH Forgiveness Intervention: A Multi-Site Randomized Controlled Trial," OSF Preprints, last edited October 20, 2023, https://osf.io/preprints/osf/8qzgw.
23. Everett Worthington, "REACH: Forgiveness of Others," Everett Worthington, accessed February 22, 2024, https://www.evworthington-forgiveness.com/reach -forgiveness-of-others.
24. "Ex-Auschwitz Guard Oskar Groening Accused of Role in 300K Deaths," NBC News, September 16, 2014, https://www.nbcnews.com/news/world/ex-auschwitz -guard-oskar-groening-accused-role-300k-deaths-n204216.
25. Jenny Stanton and Jennifer Newton, "'Forgiveness Is Free—It Is What Our World Desperately Needs': Holocaust Survivor Who Was Taken to Death Camp Aged 10 Describes Why She Hugged Her Captor the Bookkeeper of Auschwitz," *Daily Mail*, January 22, 2016, https://www.dailymail.co.uk/news/article-3412660 /Forgiveness-free-world-desperately-needs-Holocaust-survivor-taken-death-camp -aged-10-describes-hugged-captor-bookkeeper-Auschwitz.html.
26. Marina Cantacuzino, "Forgiving the Nazis Is Incomprehensible—but It Has Saved One Survivor's Life," *Guardian*, May 1, 2015, https://www.theguardian .com/commentisfree/2015/may/01/forgiving-abuse-not-forgetting-auschwitz -eva-kor.

27. Richard Goldstein, "Eva Kor, Survivor of Twin Experiments at Auschwitz, Dies at 85," *New York Times*, July 7, 2019, https://www.nytimes.com/2019/07/07/obituaries/eva-kor-dead.html.

28. Rubin Khoddam, "How Trauma Affects the Body," *Psychology Today*, March 3, 2021, https://www.psychologytoday.com/us/blog/the-addiction-connection/202103/how-trauma-affects-the-body.

29. Donald Miller, *Hero on a Mission: A Path to a Meaningful Life* (New York: HarperCollins Leadership, 2022), xiii.

30. Crystal Raypole, "How to Identify and Deal with a Victim Mentality," Healthline, updated March 15, 2023, https://www.healthline.com/health/victim-mentality.

31. Miller, *Hero on a Mission*, xiii.

32. Francis, Encyclical Letter *Laudato Si'*, Vatican, May 24, 2015, https://www.vatican.va/content/francesco/en/encyclicals/documents/papa-francesco_20150524_enciclica-laudato-si.html.

CHAPTER 9: FINDING—AND BEING—A GOOD FRIEND

1. Dan Buettner, *The Blue Zones: Lessons for Living Longer from the People Who've Lived the Longest* (Washington, DC: National Geographic, 2010).

2. "Strengthen Relationships for a Longer, Healthier Life," Harvard Health Publishing, January 18, 2011, https://www.health.harvard.edu/healthbeat/strengthen-relationships-for-longer-healthier-life.

3. Lisa F. Berkman and S. Leonard Syme, "Social Networks, Host Resistance, and Mortality: A Nine-Year Follow-up Study of Alameda County Residents," *American Journal of Epidemiology* 109, no. 2 (February 1979): 186–204, https://pubmed.ncbi.nlm.nih.gov/425958.

4. "Psychological Benefits of Friendship," WebMD, October 25, 2021, https://www.webmd.com/mental-health/psychological-benefits-of-friendship.

5. "Dunbar's Number: Why We Can Only Maintain 150 Relationships," BBC, October 9, 2019, https://www.bbc.com/future/article/20191001-dunbars-number-why-we-can-only-maintain-150-relationships.

6. For a more in-depth version of this exercise, see the challenge at the end of the chapter.

7. Rick Hellman, "How to Make Friends? Study Reveals How Many Hours It Takes," KU News, March 28, 2018, https://news.ku.edu/news/article/2018/03/06/study-reveals-number-hours-it-takes-make-friend.

8. Brené Brown, *Dare to Lead: Brave Work. Tough Conversations. Whole Hearts.* (New York: Random House, 2018), 48.

9. Géza Gergely Ambrus et al., "Getting to Know You: Emerging Neural Representations during Face Familiarization," *Journal of Neuroscience* 41, no. 26 (June 30, 2021): 5687–5698, https://www.jneurosci.org/content/41/26/5687/.

NOTES

CHAPTER 10: HARMONY AT HOME

1. Andy Cerda, "Family Time Is Far More Important Than Other Aspects of Life for Most Americans," Pew Research Center, May 26, 2023, https://www.pewresearch.org/short-reads/2023/05/26/family-time-is-far-more-important-than-other-aspects-of-life-for-most-americans/.

2. "Strong Families: What They Are, How They Work," Raising Children Network (Australia), last updated May 4, 2023, https://raisingchildren.net.au/grown-ups/family-life/routines-rituals-relationships/strong-families.

3. Kathryn Walton et al., "Exploring the Role of Family Functioning in the Association between Frequency of Family Dinners and Dietary Intake among Adolescents and Young Adults," *JAMA Network Open* 1, no. 7 (November 21, 2018): e185217, https://jamanetwork.com/journals/jamanetworkopen/fullarticle/2715616.

4. Jerica M. Berge et al., "The Protective Role of Family Meals for Youth Obesity: 10-Year Longitudinal Associations," *Journal of Pediatrics* 166, no. 2 (February 2015): 296–301, https://www.jpeds.com/article/S0022-3476%2814%2900777-X/pdf.

5. Charles Duhigg, *The Power of Habit: Why We Do What We Do and How to Change It* (New York: Random House, 2012), 109.

6. Jill Anderson, "The Benefit of Family Mealtime," Harvard Graduate School of Education, April 1, 2020, https://www.gse.harvard.edu/ideas/edcast/20/04/benefit-family-mealtime.

7. Anderson, "Benefit of Family Mealtime."

8. Becky Kennedy (Dr. Becky at Good Inside), "Our feelings don't make us good or bad people," Facebook, November 26, 2020, https://www.facebook.com/photo/?fbid=196582041962019&set=a.103672637919627.

9. Jill Bolte Taylor, *My Stroke of Insight: A Brain Scientist's Personal Journey* (New York: Penguin Books, 2016), 164.

CHAPTER 11: SABBATH

1. Missy Takano, "What Is the Sabbath in the Bible and Should Christians Observe It?," BibleProject, January 6, 2020, https://bibleproject.com/articles/keeping-the-sabbath-is-it-still-relevant-to-christians-today/.

2. Eugene H. Peterson, "The Good-for-Nothing Sabbath," April 4, 1994, *Christianity Today*, https://www.christianitytoday.com/ct/1994/april-4/good-for-nothing-sabbath.html.

3. "Findings for Longevity," Loma Linda University Health, accessed February 21, 2024, https://adventisthealthstudy.org/studies/AHS-1/findings-longevity.

4. Shayna Waltower, "50-Hour Workweeks? How to Cut Back on the New Normal," Business News Daily, October 24, 2023, https://www.businessnewsdaily.com/8357-longer-work-weeks.html.

5. Pete Grieve, "Americans Work Hundreds of Hours More a Year Than Europeans:

Report," *Money*, January 6, 2023, https://money.com/americans-work-hours-vs-europe-china/.

6. Anna Baluch, "Average PTO in the US and Other PTO Statistics (2024)," Forbes Advisor, *Forbes*, March 30, 2023, https://www.forbes.com/advisor/business/pto-statistics/.

CHAPTER 12: FINDING YOUR PURPOSE

1. Patrick L. Hill and Nicholas A. Turiano, "Purpose in Life as a Predictor of Mortality across Adulthood," *Psychological Science* 25, no. 7 (May 8, 2014): 1482–1486, https://journals.sagepub.com/doi/10.1177/0956797614531799.

2. Aaron De Smet et al., "The Great Attrition Is Making Hiring Harder. Are You Searching the Right Talent Pools?," McKinsey and Company, July 2022, https://www.mckinsey.com/capabilities/people-and-organizational-performance/our-insights/the-great-attrition-is-making-hiring-harder-are-you-searching-the-right-talent-pools.

3. Michael Lipka, "Partisans Agree: Time with Family and Friends Is Meaningful and Fulfilling," Pew Research Center, November 22, 2022, https://www.pewresearch.org/short-reads/2022/11/22/partisans-agree-time-with-family-and-friends-is-meaningful-and-fulfilling/.

4. Frederick Buechner, *Wishful Thinking: A Seeker's ABC*, rev. ed. (San Francisco: HarperSanFrancisco, 1993), 118–119.

5. Martin R. Huecker et al., "Imposter Phenomenon," StatPearls (Treasure Island, FL: StatPearls Publishing), updated July 31, 2023, https://www.ncbi.nlm.nih.gov/books/NBK585058/.

6. Ichiro Kishimi and Fumitake Koga, *The Courage to Be Disliked* (London: Allen and Unwin, 2019), 49.

ABOUT THE AUTHOR

Caroline Fausel is the owner and blogger behind Olive You Whole, a successful clean-eating and lifestyle blog. She is passionate about helping women live healthier, more intentional lives. As a health coach, she has developed a loyal community of followers who love her recipes and guidance on living a toxic-free lifestyle. Caroline is married to her college sweetheart, Chaz, and they have two precious kiddos, Ella Rae and Owen. They call Denver, Colorado, home and love hiking and skiing in the great Rocky Mountains when they're not traveling around the world.

Tyndale | REFRESH

Think Well. Live Well. Be Well.

Experience the flourishing of your mind, body, and soul with Tyndale Refresh.

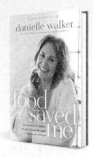
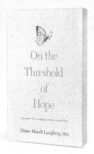
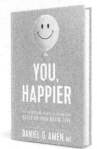
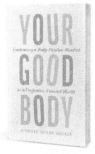

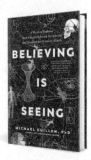
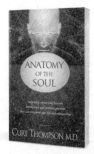
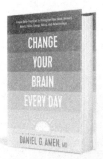
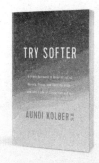

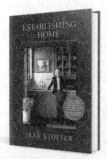
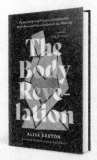
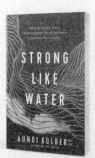
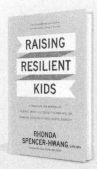

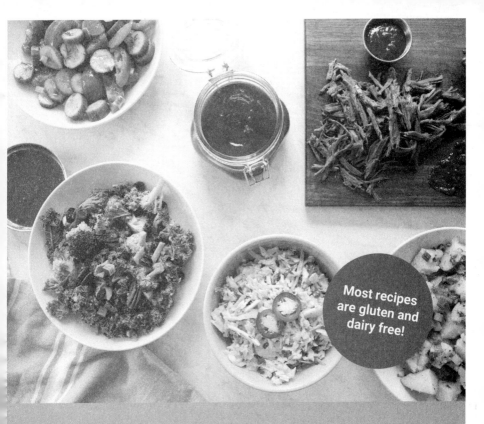

Most recipes are gluten and dairy free!

Olive You WHOLE

Our goal at Olive You Whole is to help you build a healthy, connected, and intentional life that fulfills your greatest purpose. Explore our website below to find recipes, resources, books, and health coaching that help you become your best self.

OLIVEYOUWHOLE.COM

*Food photography by Mary Britton Senseney

CP1994